WOMEN'S HEALTH THROUGH THE LENS OF *IKIGAI*

Ikigai Helps Women Gain a Sense of Purpose, Self-Confidence and Emotional Resilience to Redirect Energy to Positive Pursuits

DR. DINESH KANFADE

Disclaimer:

While the publisher and author have used their best efforts in preparing this book, they make no representation or warranties with respect to the accuracy or completeness of the contents of this book and specifically disclaim any implied warranties of merchantability or fitness for a particular purpose. No warranty may be created or extended by sales representatives or written sales materials. The advice and strategies contained herein may not be suitable for your situation. This book is for educational purpose only. It is not intended for the substitute for the diagnosis, treatment and advice of a qualified licensed professional. You should consult your healthcare provider for individualized advice. Neither the publisher nor the author shall be liable for any other commercial damages, including but not limited to special, incidental, consequential, personal, or other damage.

ACKNOWLEDGEMENTS

I wish to express my gratitude to various sources, knowingly or unknowingly has contributed for empowering my knowledge, empowering women's health and helping me to write this book.

I would like to thank my mentors and teachers who had been a torch bearer for me for writing this book.

I am extremely thankful to **Dr. Girija Wagh, Professor, Dept. of OBGYN Bharti Vidyapeeth Medical College Hospital, Pune** for taking time from her busy schedule to write **"FOREWORD"** for my book.

Book images Credit and Courtesy: *

Diagrammatic representation of Ikigai

Source: By en: User: Nimbosa derived from works
File: Ikigai-En-svg-Wikimedia Commons

https://commons.wikimedia.org/wiki/File:Ikigai-EN.svg#/media/File:Ikigai-EN.svg

I also express my sincere gratitude to my family members and friends who have always been supportive and motivated me in my initiatives in writing series of books on **"Women's Health"**, this book being 11th in the series.

DEDICATION

Dedicated to my better half Nita,

son Akshay, daughter-in-law Priya

and little sweet Avni.

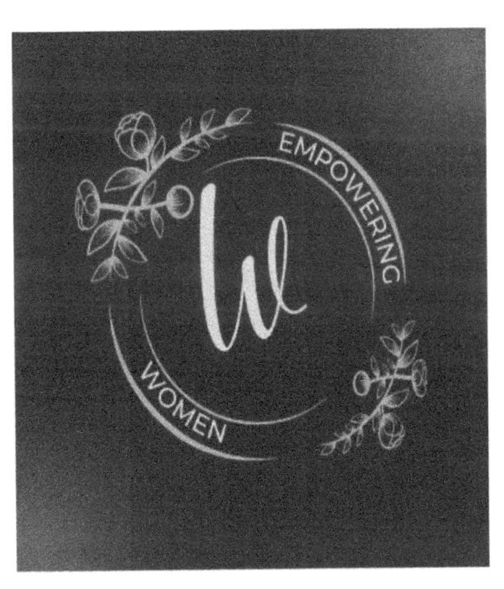

EMPOWERING
WOMEN

"It is the woman who should be awakened first.

Once she is on the move,

the family moves, the village moves,

and ultimately the nation moves."

-Pandit Jawaharlal Nehru

"Ikigai is not about being perfect. It's about discovering your purpose, overcoming challenges, and making better choices about your health."

-Anonymous

FOREWORD

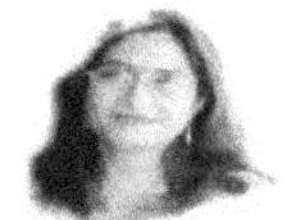

Dr.Girija Wagh

It is an absolute honor to write the foreword for ***Women's Health Through the Lens of Ikigai,*** a book that seamlessly integrates medical science with the timeless wisdom of purposeful living. In a world where women often prioritize the needs of others before their own, this book serves as a gentle yet powerful reminder that self-care is not a luxury but a necessity.

The author, with years of experience as a gynecologist, has thoughtfully crafted a guide that speaks to every woman—whether she is navigating adolescence, embracing motherhood, or transitioning through menopause. By incorporating the principles of ***Ikigai***, this book provides not only medical insights but also an inspiring framework for aligning health with life's deeper purpose.

What sets this book apart is its ability to transform the way we perceive women's health. It encourages readers to move beyond routine check-ups and fitness regimens, fostering a mindset where well-being is deeply connected to joy, fulfillment, and meaning. It challenges the traditional notions of health and offers a revolutionary perspective—one that is both enlightening and empowering.

I am confident that the book ***"Women's Health Through the Lens of Ikigai"*** will resonate with readers, offering them practical wisdom and motivation to take charge of their health in a holistic and meaningful way. This book is not just a guide—it is a movement towards redefining women's health with grace, intention, and purpose.

With admiration and best wishes,

DR. GIRIJA WAGH

MD, FICOG, DIP ENDO, FICS.

- **Obstetrician / Gynecologist & IVF Specialist.**
- **Professor, Dept. of OBGYN** Bharti Vidyapeeth Medical College Hospital, Pune.
- **Sr. Consultant,** Cloud Nine & Apollo Hospital Pune.
- **Elected Vice President FOGSI** West Zone, 2024.
- **Faculty Professor**, OGASH International Experts General Coordinator (2016).
- **Chairman, Medical Disorders in Pregnancy Committee** FOGSI (2012 – 2016).
- **Vice President,** India Chapter Gestosis (since 2014).
- **Member**, Central Supervisory Board of the **PCPNDT Act** (2010 – 2014).
- **Assistant Coordinator, National Eclampsia Registry** (since 2008).
- **National Mentor**, LAQSHYA-NPOQCN, MOHFW, GOI.
- **Peer Reviewer:** JOGI, BJOG, EJOG.
- **Regional Director** StudyMedic.
- **Anandibai Joshi Award** for Excellence in Medical Services.

PREFACE

Health is a journey, not a destination. As a gynecologist, I have spent years guiding women through various stages of life—adolescence, motherhood, and menopause—witnessing firsthand the intricate interplay between physical well-being, mental resilience, and emotional balance. Over the time, I realized that traditional medical advice often addresses symptoms but rarely explores the deeper motivations that drive a woman's commitment to her own health. This realization led me to discover the profound wisdom of *Ikigai*, the Japanese philosophy of finding purpose and meaning in life.

The concept of *Ikigai* beautifully aligns with the unique challenges and aspirations of women. It is not merely about longevity but about living a life filled with joy, fulfillment, and balance. When applied to health, *Ikigai* transforms the conventional approach to well-being, moving beyond diet charts and exercise routines to integrate a deeper sense of purpose, connection, and self-care into daily life.

This book, ***Women's Health Through the Lens of Ikigai***, is an attempt to bridge the gap between medical science and the philosophy of purposeful living. It is designed to empower women to take charge of their health with a holistic approach—one that nurtures the body, mind, and soul. Through the lens of Ikigai, we will explore how women can align their health goals with their passions, values, and life's purpose, creating a sustainable and joyful path to wellness.

Each chapter delves into different phases of a woman's life, offering insights into how Ikigai can be a guiding force during hormonal transitions, reproductive health challenges, and the evolving dynamics of aging. The book also addresses the often-overlooked emotional and psychological aspects of health, emphasizing self-care as a necessity rather than a luxury.

I hope that this book serves as a companion to every woman seeking balance, vitality, and meaning in her health journey. May it inspire you to embrace wellness not as an obligation but as an integral part of a fulfilling life.

With warmth and gratitude,

DR. DINESH KANFADE

MBBS., DGO., DFP., FICMCH., CIMP.

Sr. Obstetrician & Gynecologist

TABLE OF CONTENT

CHAPTER I: INTRODUCTION

"When women are healthy, families flourish,

Communities grow, and nations thrive."

- Anonymous

(A) Definition of Ikigai, It's Origin and Overview

Definition of Ikigai:

Ikigai is a Japanese concept that refers to the reason for being or the thing that gives one's life meaning and purpose. It is often seen as the intersection of four key elements:

1. What you love (your passion).
2. What you are good at (your profession or talent).
3. What the world needs (your mission or contribution).
4. What you can be paid for (your vocation or livelihood).

The word suggests a deep sense of satisfaction and fulfillment that comes from living a meaningful life aligned with one's values and passions.

Etymology and Origin of Ikigai:

The term **ikigai (生き甲斐)** is derived from two Japanese words:

Iki (生き): Meaning "life" or "to live."

Gai (甲斐): Meaning "worth," "value," or "benefit."

The **suffix "gai"** comes from the word **kai**, which means "shell" in Japanese. In ancient Japan, shells were considered highly valuable, symbolizing something precious or worthwhile. Over time, "gai" evolved to represent things of value, thus combining to form *Ikigai*, which means "a reason for living" or "something that makes life worthwhile."

Origin and Cultural Background:

The concept of *Ikigai* is deeply rooted in Japanese culture and philosophy. It has been an intrinsic part of Japanese life for centuries and is particularly associated with the longevity and happiness of people living in Okinawa, a region known for its high percentage of centenarians. For the Okinawans, *Ikigai* is not just a philosophical idea but a practical way of life, often linked to strong social ties, healthy living, and purposeful activity.

Ikigai is not confined to large, life-changing goals; it can also encompass small joys and routines, such as gardening, cooking, or spending time with loved ones. In Japanese culture, *Ikigai* is about balancing life's small pleasures and long-term goals.

Overview of Ikigai:

At its core, *Ikigai* reflects the idea that happiness and fulfillment come from finding harmony between personal and societal needs. While the Western interpretation often visualizes *Ikigai* as the intersection of four circles (passion, mission, vocation, and profession), the traditional Japanese view is more subtle and personalized. It does not always emphasize monetary gain or professional success but instead focuses on what makes life worth living on an individual level.

Key aspects of ikigai:

1. **Purpose-driven life:** Aligning daily actions with one's values and goals.

2. **Balance and moderation:** Living a life that incorporates work, leisure, and relationships.

3. **Connection with community:** Building strong bonds with family, friends, and society.

4. **Health and longevity:** Maintaining physical, mental, and emotional well-being.

Modern Relevance: *Ikigai* has gained global recognition as a tool for achieving personal and professional fulfillment. It encourages people to reflect on their purpose, identify their unique gifts, and align their activities with their passions and values. This makes it a universal concept that transcends cultural boundaries while retaining its Japanese origins.

(B) Importance of Women's Health in General

Women's health is a cornerstone of societal well-being, as women play critical roles in families, communities, and the workforce. Prioritizing women's health is essential not only for their personal well-being but also for fostering healthy families, sustainable societies, and economic development.

Below are key reasons why women's health is crucial:

1. Foundation of Family and Community Health

- Women often act as caregivers, nurturing children, spouses, and elderly family members. A healthy woman ensures better care for others.

- Maternal health impacts the health and survival of children. Proper prenatal care, nutrition, and safe childbirth reduce infant mortality rates and improve family health.

- Educated and healthy women are more likely to make informed decisions about family planning, nutrition, and health care for their families.

2. Economic and Societal Impact

- Women constitute nearly half of the global workforce. Healthy women contribute to economic growth and productivity.

- Unhealthy women often face reduced workforce participation, leading to economic losses both for families and society.

- Empowering women with good health ensures gender equality in education, employment, and leadership roles.

3. Unique Health Needs

Women experience unique biological and hormonal changes throughout their lives, such as:

- **Menstruation**: Menstrual health is critical for overall well-being, as conditions like irregular periods, PCOS, and anemia can affect physical and emotional health.

- **Pregnancy and Maternal Health**: Proper care during pregnancy ensures the health of both mother and baby, reducing the risks of complications such as gestational diabetes or preeclampsia.

- **Menopause**: Supporting women during menopause prevents issues like osteoporosis, cardiovascular problems, and emotional distress.

4. Prevention of Chronic Diseases

Women are at a higher risk for certain diseases, such as:

- **Breast and Cervical Cancer**: Regular screenings like mammograms and Pap smears can save lives through early detection.

- **Heart Disease**: Although often considered a "male" issue, heart disease is the leading cause of death in women. Awareness and prevention are crucial.

- **Osteoporosis**: Women are more prone to bone loss due to hormonal changes during menopause, making early prevention and treatment important.

5. Mental and Emotional Health

- Women are more likely to experience depression, anxiety, and postpartum mood disorders due to biological, social, and cultural factors.

- Promoting emotional well-being through mental health support and stress management is essential for maintaining overall health.

6. Reproductive and Sexual Health

- Access to safe and informed reproductive health care is a fundamental right for women.

- Education about contraception, family planning, and sexually transmitted diseases (STDs) can empower women to make better health decisions.

- Preventing and managing reproductive health issues like endometriosis, infertility, and uterine fibroids are vital for a woman's quality of life.

7. Gender Equality and Empowerment

- When women have access to quality health care, they are better able to participate in education, careers, and leadership roles, promoting gender equality.

- Healthy women are more likely to advocate for their rights and take on leadership positions, fostering progress in their communities.

8. Health Across Life Stages

Women's health needs vary significantly at different stages of life:

- **Adolescence**: Proper education about puberty, menstrual hygiene, and mental health is vital for young girls.

- **Reproductive Age**: Care during pregnancy, childbirth, and lactation ensures a healthy transition into motherhood.

- **Menopause and Aging**: Supporting women during menopause reduces the risk of chronic conditions like osteoporosis, heart disease, and mental health issues.

9. Breaking Generational Cycles

- Healthy women ensure healthy children, breaking the cycle of malnutrition, poor health, and poverty.

- Educated mothers are more likely to raise educated children, contributing to the development of future generations.

10. Global Health Goals

- Women's health is a priority in global health initiatives like the United Nations' Sustainable Development Goals (SDGs), particularly Goal 3 (Good Health and Well-being) and Goal 5 (Gender Equality).

- Addressing women's health issues ensures progress toward universal health care, reducing maternal mortality, and achieving gender equity.

In summary, women's health is not just a personal issue; it is a societal, economic, and global concern. By prioritizing women's health through access to quality care, education, and empowerment, we can create healthier families, stronger communities, and a more equitable world.

(C) Analysis of the Statement of Pandit Jawaharlal Nehru: First Prime Minister of India

Pandit Jawaharlal Nehru's statement, **"It is the woman who should be awakened first. Once she is on the move, the family moves, the village moves and ultimately the nation moves,"** beautifully encapsulates the central role of women in shaping families, communities, and nations. Let's analyze and comment on its deeper significance:

1. Women as Catalysts of Change

- Nehru recognized the pivotal role women play in societal progress. Empowering women is not an isolated action—it has a multiplier effect.

- When women are educated, empowered, and given opportunities, they drive transformations in their families, setting an example and raising a generation of well-informed and capable individuals.

- Women's involvement in social, economic, and political spheres accelerates national development as they bring unique perspectives and skills.

2. The Role of Women in Families

- Women are often the first educators and caretakers in families. When a woman is "awakened" through education, awareness, and empowerment, her influence uplifts not just herself but also her children and extended family.

- An educated mother ensures her children receive education, proper nutrition, and values, breaking the cycle of poverty and ignorance.

- In families, women often act as mediators, caregivers, and managers, making them key to fostering unity and progress.

3. Community and Village Development

- Women's participation in villages, especially in rural India, has a profound impact on grassroots development. Initiatives like **self-help groups (SHGs)** and rural entrepreneurship demonstrate how women drive economic and social change.

- Empowered women take active roles in community decisions, advocate for education, health, and infrastructure, and ensure inclusive progress at the village level.

- Examples include women sarpanches (village heads) and leaders of rural development programs, whose efforts have led to tangible improvements in sanitation, education, and healthcare.

4. National Progress and Economic Growth

- At a national level, the participation of women in the workforce boosts the economy. Research shows that gender equality in labor markets can significantly increase a country's GDP.

- Women's representation in politics, governance, and leadership strengthens democracies and ensures more inclusive policies.

- Nehru's emphasis on women's awakening resonates today, as nations worldwide recognize the role of gender equality in achieving sustainable development goals (SDGs).

5. Historical Context of Nehru's Vision

- Nehru's statement was made in post-independence India, a time when women faced severe social, educational, and economic inequalities.

- He foresaw that for India to prosper, half its population (women) had to be uplifted. Education and empowerment of women were seen as key to eradicating regressive practices like child marriage, dowry, and gender discrimination.

- His vision is reflected in modern India's strides in women's empowerment through policies, education programs, and representation in various sectors.

6. Modern Relevance

- In today's world, Nehru's statement remains deeply relevant. Challenges like gender inequality, illiteracy, and lack of healthcare access still disproportionately affect women, especially in rural and underprivileged areas.

- **Narendra Modi Government** has realized the importance of women's empowerment and launched several schemes aimed at empowering women across various sectors. Here are some initiatives:

- **"Beti Bachao Beti Padhao"** (Save the daughter, Educate the daughter) is a flagship initiative launched by the Government of India in 2015 to address declining child sex ratio and promote girls' education. The campaign focuses on three main areas:

  - **Prevention of Gender-Based Sex Selection** – Addressing the deep-routed issue of female feticide and ensuring strict implementation of the **PCPNDT Act** (Pre-Conception and Pre-Natal Diagnostic Techniques Act).

- o **Ensuring Survival and Protection of the Girl Child** – Promoting better healthcare, nutrition and empower them for a brighter future.

- o **Promoting Education and Participation** – Encouraging families to educate girls and empower them for a brighter future.

- **Pradhan Mantri Matru Vandana Yojana (PMMVY)** – A maternity benefit scheme providing financial assistance to pregnant and lactating mothers for their first child.

- **Ujjwala Yojana** – Provides free LPG connections to women from poor households to reduce health hazards from traditional cooking fuels.

- **Sukanya Samruddhi Yojana (SSY)** – A savings scheme under Beti Bachao Beti Padhao to secure the future of the girl child.

- **Poshan Abhiyan** – A nutrition scheme focusing on reducing malnutrition among women, pregnant mothers, and children.

- **MUDRA Yojana** – Provides collateral-free loans to women entrepreneurs to promote self-employment and small businesses.

- **Mission Shakti** – A comprehensive initiative for women's safety, security, and empowerment, integrating existing schemes like Beti Bachao Beti Padhao and One Stop Centers.

In summary, Nehru's words are a timeless reminder that true progress begins with empowering women.

As the saying goes,

"When you educate a woman, you educate a generation."

Changes in Population Structure in India in Coming Years: Need for Awareness and Training

- ✓ The current life expectancy for India is 70.82 years, a 0.29% increase in 2024.
- ✓ By 2046, the elderly population in India is projected to surpass the population of 0 – 14 years – **UNFPA** India.
- ✓ By 2050, older population will be 20.6% of total population.
- ✓ From 2022 to 2050, older population will grow by 134%.
- ✓ Today, most women spend more than one-third of their lives after menopause.
- ✓ Life expectancy for a woman at 60 years of age is 19 years, while for men it is 17.5 years.
- ✓ *Significant changes in age and gender structure are being observed, it is going to be the feminization of elderly population in years to come and hinting us to be prepared for the challenges.*

(D) Relevance of Ikigai to Women's Health and Well-being

The concept of *Ikigai*—finding one's purpose and meaning in life—has significant relevance to women's health and well-being. Women face unique challenges at different stages of life, such as adolescence, motherhood, menopause, and beyond, which impact both physical and emotional health. By applying the principles of *Ikigai*, women can create a more balanced, fulfilling, and healthy life.

1. Emotional Well-being and Mental Health

- **Stress Reduction**: Identifying a purpose can help women manage stress by focusing on what truly matters to them.

- **Sense of Fulfillment**: Living aligned with their *Ikigai* fosters a sense of accomplishment, reducing anxiety, depression, and feelings of being overwhelmed.

- **Self-awareness**: Exploring *Ikigai* promotes self-reflection, helping women better understand their needs, passions, and values, which are essential for emotional resilience.

2. Physical Health and Longevity

- **Healthy Lifestyle Choices**: *Ikigai* encourages women to pursue activities they enjoy and that contribute to their health, such as yoga, walking, or preparing nutritious meals.

- **Hormonal Health**: Stress and emotional imbalance can exacerbate hormonal changes during menstruation, pregnancy, and menopause. Focusing on *Ikigai* can help regulate stress-related health issues like PCOS, thyroid disorders, and menopause symptoms.

- **Enhanced Longevity**: As observed in Okinawan women, having a clear sense of purpose is correlated with better health and longer life expectancy.

3. Reproductive and Maternal Health

- **Navigating Motherhood**: For mothers, *Ikigai* can help balance caregiving responsibilities with personal goals, reducing burnout and promoting mental clarity.

- **Postpartum Well-being**: Finding purpose beyond the role of motherhood can aid in overcoming postpartum depression and maintaining a sense of identity.

- **Body Positivity**: *Ikigai* promotes acceptance and appreciation of one's body, fostering confidence and reducing societal pressures related to physical appearance.

4. Menopause and Aging

- **Coping with Life Transitions**: *Ikigai* helps women embrace menopause and aging as natural phases of life, rather than as losses of youth.

- **Rediscovering Purpose**: Many women struggle with an "empty nest" syndrome or identity shifts post-menopause. *Ikigai* encourages exploring new passions, hobbies, and career paths.

- **Maintaining Social Bonds**: The sense of community emphasized in *ikigai* can reduce feelings of loneliness and isolation, which are common during later stages of life.

5. Work-Life Balance

- **Career Fulfillment**: By aligning professional goals with *Ikigai*, women can experience satisfaction in their work without feeling disconnected or overburdened.

- **Balancing Roles**: *Ikigai* provides a framework to harmonize personal and professional roles, ensuring neither dominates at the cost of health or happiness.

6. Enhancing Relationships

- **Building Stronger Bonds**: *Ikigai* emphasizes meaningful connections with others, which can lead to better relationships with family, friends, and partners.

- **Empathy and Support**: Purpose-driven living encourages emotional availability, which strengthens familial and social ties.

7. Resilience During Challenges

- **Handling Life's Struggles**: *Ikigai* serves as an anchor during hardships, whether they arise from health issues, caregiving responsibilities, or societal expectations.

- **Inner Strength**: By focusing on what gives life meaning, women can cultivate emotional resilience and a positive outlook even during difficult times.

8. Holistic Well-being

- **Mind-Body Connection**: *Ikigai* aligns with practices like mindfulness, meditation, and self-care, which promote overall well-being.

- **Alignment with Natural Rhythms**: *Ikigai* encourages women to honor their biological and emotional cycles, fostering self-compassion and a deeper connection with their health.

In summary, Ikigai offers women a holistic approach to well-being by addressing the interplay of emotional, physical, and social health. It empowers women to live purposefully through all stages of life, navigate challenges with resilience, and maintain harmony between their personal and professional identities. By integrating Ikigai into daily life, women can cultivate a more balanced, healthy, and fulfilling existence.

(E) Objectives and Target Audience of my Book

Objectives of the Book

- **Introduce the Concept of *Ikigai:***
  - Explain the philosophy of *Ikigai* and how it applies to women's lives at different stages.

  - Help women identify their personal *Ikigai* to lead a purposeful and fulfilling life.

- **Promote Holistic Well-being:**
  - Illustrate how aligning the four pillars of *Ikigai* contributes to physical, emotional, and mental health.

  - Provide actionable insights for achieving balance and happiness.

- **Empower Women Through Self-Discovery:**
  - Offer tools, strategies, and examples for women to explore their passions, talents, and purpose.

  - Encourage women to embrace their individuality while navigating life's challenges.

- **Enhance Health Awareness:**
  - Highlight the connection between purpose-driven living and improved physical health, mental resilience, and longevity.

  - Provide practical guidance for incorporating healthy habits into daily life.

- **Address Women's Unique Health Challenges:**
  - Discuss health concerns specific to women, such as hormonal health, reproductive well-being, and

menopause, and how *Ikigai* can help manage these phases.

  - o Offer solutions for overcoming stress, burnout, and societal pressures.

- **Inspire Societal Change**:
  - o Advocate for a cultural shift in how women's health and purpose are perceived and supported.

  - o Empower readers to become change-makers in their communities by leading purposeful lives.

Target Audience

- **Women Across Life Stages**:
  - o Adolescents and young women exploring identity and purpose.

  - o Working professionals juggling careers and personal responsibilities.

  - o Mothers seeking balance between caregiving and self-fulfillment.

  - o Women in menopause or retirement rediscovering purpose and vitality.

- **Health and Wellness Enthusiasts**:
  - o Women interested in holistic health practices, mental well-being, and mindfulness.

  - o Individuals looking for practical ways to integrate purpose with well-being.

- **Professionals in Health and Education**:
  - o Gynecologists, psychologists, and wellness coaches who want to understand how *Ikigai* can support women's health.

  - o Educators and mentors working to empower women.

- **Caregivers and Advocates**:
  - o Family members, friends, and community leaders looking to support women in their journey toward health and happiness.

- **Readers Interested in Self-Improvement**:
  - o Anyone seeking inspiration and actionable advice for living a balanced, purposeful, and fulfilling life, especially through the lens of women's experiences.

CHAPTER II: UNDERSTANDING IKIGAI

"Ikigai is the art of living with balance—

doing what you love, what the world needs,

and what brings you inner peace."

-Anonymous

(A) Concept of Ikegai

The concept of *Ikigai* revolves around the harmonious intersection of four key pillars, which together guide an individual toward a purposeful and fulfilling life. These pillars represent different dimensions of life and help balance personal passions with societal needs. Let's delve into each pillar:

1. What You Love (Passion)

- This pillar is about identifying activities and pursuits that bring you joy and fulfillment. It reflects the things you naturally enjoy doing without external motivation.

- It aligns with your inner passions and emotional satisfaction.

- Examples: Playing an instrument, painting, gardening, mentoring, or traveling.

Key Question: What activities make you lose track of time and feel alive?

2. What You Are Good At (Profession)

- This pillar focuses on your skills, talents, and expertise—things you excel at and have developed over time through education, training, or natural ability.

- It encourages you to identify your strengths and leverage them in ways that make a meaningful impact.

- Examples: Writing, teaching, coding, designing, or problem-solving.

Key Question: What are you skilled at or naturally talented in?

3. What the World Needs (Mission)

- This pillar connects your purpose to the greater good by identifying how your skills and passions can contribute to society.

- It emphasizes aligning your goals with the needs of your community, environment, or the world at large.

- Examples: Addressing social issues, creating solutions for underserved populations, or contributing to sustainable living.

Key Question: How can your efforts make a positive difference in the world?

4. What You Can Be Paid For (Vocation)

- This pillar highlights the practical aspect of earning a livelihood while pursuing your passion and mission.

- It encourages you to explore ways to monetize your talents and passions sustainably.

- Examples: Freelancing, starting a business, offering consulting services, or pursuing a professional career.

Key Question: What services or skills can you offer that people are willing to pay for?

The Intersections of the Four Pillars

When these four pillars overlap, they create distinct areas of meaning:

- **Passion**: Where "What You Love" and "What You Are Good At" intersect.

- **Mission**: Where "What You Love" and "What the World Needs" intersect.

- **Vocation**: Where "What the World Needs" and "What You Can Be Paid For" intersect.

- **Profession**: Where "What You Are Good At" and "What You Can Be Paid For" intersect.

Ikigai: The Center of Balance

True *Ikigai* lies at the center, where all four pillars converge. It represents a life in which:

- You are doing something you love.

- You are skilled and competent in it.

- It fulfills a meaningful purpose for others.

- It provides financial stability or rewards.

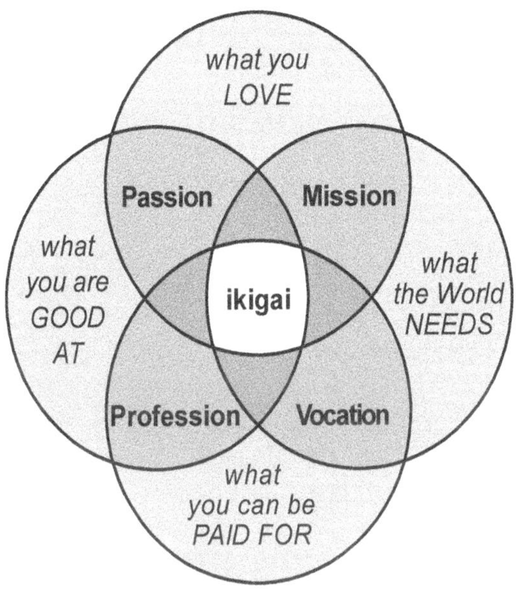

Source: By en: User: Nimbosa derived from works File: Ikigai-En-svg-Wikimedia Commons

https://commons.wikimedia.org/wiki/File:Ikigai-EN.svg#/media/File:Ikigai-EN.svg

By balancing these pillars, individuals can find purpose, achieve personal and professional fulfillment, and contribute to society while living a satisfying and harmonious life.

In summary, the four pillars of Ikigai provide a framework to explore life's meaning and purpose, guiding individuals toward a balanced and joyful existence. By reflecting on each pillar, you can align your passions, skills, societal contributions, and financial needs to live a life of fulfillment and impact.

(B) How the Four Pillars of Ikigai Can Shape Women's Overall Health and Happiness

The four pillars of *Ikigai*—**What You Love**, **What You Are Good At**, **What the World Needs**, and **What You Can Be Paid For**—can significantly contribute to women's overall health and happiness by fostering a sense of balance, purpose, and fulfillment. Here's how each pillar impacts women's well-being:

1. What You Love (Passion): Emotional and Mental Health

- **Impact on Health**: Engaging in activities you love enhances emotional well-being, reduces stress, and fosters mental clarity. Whether it's a hobby like painting, dancing, or gardening, it can act as a therapeutic outlet for emotions.

- **Impact on Happiness**: Doing what you love creates joy and fulfillment, combating feelings of monotony or burnout. For women balancing multiple roles, indulging in passions can provide an escape and restore emotional balance.

- **Example**: A mother passionate about yoga finds a personal space to rejuvenate, which improves her mood and resilience in daily life.

Key Connection to Health*: Passion activities lower cortisol levels, reduce anxiety, and promote happiness.*

2. What You Are Good At (Profession): Confidence and Personal Growth

- **Impact on Health**: Recognizing and honing one's skills boosts self-esteem, which is vital for mental health. It also prevents feelings of inadequacy and helps combat societal pressures to "do it all."

- **Impact on Happiness**: Acknowledging and developing talents can lead to a sense of accomplishment. It empowers women to take pride in their individuality and contributions, fostering long-term happiness.

- **Example**: A woman skilled in baking who starts a small bakery feels more confident, financially independent, and valued for her abilities.

Key Connection to Health: *Personal growth boosts dopamine levels, improving overall well-being and combating mental health challenges like depression.*

3. What the World Needs (Mission): Social Connection and Purpose

- **Impact on Health**: Contributing to the well-being of others builds a sense of purpose, which has been shown to improve physical health and increase longevity. Women who feel they are making a difference are often more motivated to stay healthy and active.

- **Impact on Happiness**: Feeling connected to a greater cause enhances life satisfaction. Women involved in meaningful missions (e.g., mentoring, volunteering, or social activism) experience a sense of fulfillment and joy.

- **Example**: A woman volunteering at a shelter for women and children finds her life enriched through meaningful social connections and the knowledge that she's helping others.

Key Connection to Health: *Purpose-driven living reduces stress hormones, boosts immunity, and creates a sense of belonging.*

4. What You Can Be Paid For (Vocation): Financial Security and Independence

- **Impact on Health**: Financial independence is directly tied to reduced stress and improved mental health. Women who can earn through their skills and passions feel empowered and are better equipped to access health care, nutrition, and wellness opportunities.

- **Impact on Happiness**: Earning through something you enjoy fosters satisfaction and eliminates the emotional strain of doing unfulfilling work. It also provides the resources to invest in personal growth, leisure, and self-care.

- **Example**: A woman passionate about writing who monetizes her skill by publishing books or freelance blogging experiences a blend of joy and financial security.

Key Connection to Health: *Financial stability lowers anxiety, provides access to better health care, and allows for self-care investments.*

The Holistic Impact of Ikigai on Women's Health and Happiness

When all four pillars converge, women experience **holistic well-being** that encompasses physical, mental, emotional, and social health:

- **Reduced Stress**: Living a purpose-driven life lowers stress levels, reducing the risk of stress-related illnesses like hypertension, diabetes, and hormonal imbalances.

- **Improved Relationships**: A woman aligned with her *Ikigai* often builds stronger relationships, as she feels fulfilled and emotionally balanced.

- **Physical Fitness**: Women motivated by their *Ikigai* are more likely to maintain a healthy lifestyle, as they see health as a tool to fulfill their purpose.

- **Resilience**: Purpose-driven women can better navigate challenges like societal expectations, career pressures, or family responsibilities.

- **Life Satisfaction**: Living with intention brings a sense of joy, gratitude, and contentment.

In summary, the four pillars of Ikigai are a transformative framework for women to achieve a balanced, purposeful, and healthy life. By aligning their passions, skills, contributions, and financial needs, women can overcome stress, enhance happiness, and foster overall well-being. In a world where women often juggle multiple roles, finding their Ikigai ensures that they thrive—not just survive.

(C) Scientific Evidence Linking Purpose to Improved Physical and Mental Health

A growing body of scientific research highlights the profound link between having a sense of purpose and improved physical and mental health. Studies suggest that purpose-driven living positively influences biological, psychological, and social well-being. Below are key findings from scientific studies:

1. Physical Health Benefits

- **Reduced Risk of Chronic Diseases**
  - **Evidence**: A 2019 study published in *JAMA Network Open* found that individuals with a higher sense of purpose were 19% less likely to die from heart, circulatory, or blood conditions.

  - **Explanation**: *Purposeful living helps regulate stress, which reduces the risk of hypertension, heart disease, and inflammation—key contributors to chronic illnesses.*

- **Longevity**
  - **Evidence**: A long-term study of over 6,000 adults from the *Journal of Psychosomatic Research* (2016) revealed that individuals with a strong sense of purpose were more likely to live longer, independent of other factors like income, education, or physical health.

  - **Explanation**: *A sense of purpose motivates people to adopt healthier lifestyles, maintain regular physical activity, and seek timely medical care.*

- **Better Sleep Quality**
  - **Evidence**: A 2017 study in *Sleep Science and Practice* reported that older adults with a higher sense of purpose experienced better sleep quality

and were less likely to suffer from sleep disorders such as insomnia.

- o **Explanation**: *Purpose reduces mental restlessness and anxiety, leading to better sleep.*

- **Improved Immune Function**
  - o **Evidence**: Research published in *Proceedings of the National Academy of Sciences* (2013) found that individuals with a strong sense of purpose had lower levels of pro-inflammatory gene expression, indicating better immune regulation.

  - o **Explanation**: *Reduced stress and greater emotional well-being enhance the body's immune response.*

2. Mental Health Benefits

- **Lower Risk of Depression and Anxiety**
  - o **Evidence**: A study in *The Lancet Psychiatry* (2019) found that people with a sense of purpose were less likely to suffer from depression, particularly in later life.

  - o **Explanation**: *Purposeful living provides a framework for meaning, which counteracts feelings of emptiness, hopelessness, and anxiety.*

- **Greater Emotional Resilience**
  - o **Evidence**: A 2014 study in *Psychological Science* showed that people with a clear purpose recover faster from emotional distress and are better equipped to cope with setbacks.

  - o **Explanation**: *Purpose fosters optimism and a forward-looking mindset, making individuals more resilient to adversity.*

- **Enhanced Cognitive Function**
  - **Evidence**: Research from *Alzheimer's & Dementia* (2012) found that older adults with a sense of purpose showed a slower rate of cognitive decline and were less likely to develop Alzheimer's disease.

  - **Explanation**: *Purpose engages the brain in goal-directed activities, promoting mental agility and reducing cognitive aging.*

- **Increased Happiness and Life Satisfaction**
  - **Evidence**: A study published in the *Journal of Positive Psychology* (2018) found that individuals with a sense of purpose reported significantly higher levels of happiness, satisfaction, and self-worth.

  - **Explanation**: *Purpose drives meaningful activities and social connections, which are integral to emotional well-being.*

3. Behavioral Health and Lifestyle Choices

- **Greater Engagement in Healthy Behaviors**
  - **Evidence**: A 2015 study in *Health Psychology* revealed that individuals with a strong sense of purpose were more likely to engage in regular physical activity, eat nutritious foods, and avoid risky behaviors like smoking or excessive alcohol consumption.

  - **Explanation**: *Purposeful people are motivated to maintain their health to achieve their life goals.*

- **Reduced Risk of Substance Abuse**
  - **Evidence**: Research in *Addiction Research & Theory* (2020) suggests that people with a clear

purpose are less likely to engage in substance abuse or addictive behaviors.

- o **Explanation**: *Purpose offers intrinsic motivation and emotional stability, reducing the need for external coping mechanisms.*

4. Social and Relational Benefits

- **Stronger Social Connections**
  - o **Evidence**: A study in *Social Science & Medicine* (2016) showed that people with purpose tend to form stronger and more meaningful relationships.

  - o **Explanation**: *Purpose promotes empathy, a sense of belonging, and the ability to build supportive social networks.*

- **Reduced Feelings of Loneliness**
  - o **Evidence**: Research published in *Aging & Mental Health* (2020) found that older adults with a sense of purpose were less likely to feel lonely, even if they lived alone.

  - o **Explanation**: *Purpose drives social engagement and gives individuals a reason to connect with others.*

5. Neuroscience of Purpose

- **Brain Activation**: Neuroscientific studies indicate that purposeful activities activate the brain's reward system, particularly the release of dopamine, which contributes to feelings of happiness and motivation.

- **Prefrontal Cortex Engagement**: Purpose-oriented individuals show increased activity in the prefrontal cortex, the area associated with decision-making, goal-setting, and emotional regulation.

In summary, scientific evidence overwhelmingly supports the link between purpose and improved physical and mental health. Purpose-driven individuals tend to live longer, experience better emotional resilience, and adopt healthier lifestyles. By providing meaning and direction, purpose serves as a powerful tool for holistic well-being, benefiting not just individuals but also their families and communities. Cultivating a sense of purpose is therefore not only a personal endeavor but a societal investment in overall health and happiness.

(D) 10 Principles of Ikigai for Women's Health

The concept of *Ikigai* originates from Japan and represents a reason for being – a deep sense of purpose that brings fulfillment and joy. Inspired by *the lifestyle of Okinawans*, who are known for their longevity and well-being; following 10 principles can be applied for "Women's Health in all stages – adolescence, reproductive life and menopause *to increase longevity and making women free from diseases,* physically as well as mentally, also living a *satisfying and harmonious life with some purpose.*

1. Embrace Lifelong Vitality:

Staying active physically and mentally at every stage of life, from adolescence to menopause, supports longevity and well-being.

2. Find Balance and Slow Down:

Managing stress, avoiding burnout, and creating space for self-care are essential for hormonal balance and overall health.

3. Nourish Your Body with Awareness:

Practicing mindful eating (similar to the 80% rule) helps regulate hormones, supports reproductive health, and reduces disease risk including PCOS or menopausal symptoms.

4. Cultivate Meaningful Connections:

Strong relationships with family, friends, and community enhance emotional resilience and mental well-being.

5. Prioritize Movement of Strength:

Engaging in regular physical activity, whether gentle (like yoga) or active (like strength training), keeps bone strong, metabolism steady and mood balanced.

6. Nurture a Positive Mindset:

A hopeful, optimistic outlook influences mental and physical health, reducing stress-related illnesses and enhancing emotional well-being.

7. Reconnect with Nature's Healing Power:

Spending time outdoors benefits mental clarity, stress management, and hormonal regulation, particularly in menopause and fertility health.

8. Practice Gratitude for Inner Harmony:

Acknowledging life's blessings enhances emotional well-being, reduces stress, and fosters resilience in times of change.

9. Be Present in Your Journey:

Whether navigating adolescence, motherhood, or aging, focusing on the present moment reduces anxiety and promotes overall well-being.

10. Discover and Live Your Purpose:

Engaging in fulfilling activities, whether in career, caregiving, or personal passions, nurtures a sense of meaning and contributes to long-term health.

(E) The Longevity of Okinawan Women: Genetics, Lifestyle, and Health

Okinawan women have long been celebrated for their remarkable longevity, with many living beyond 100 years while maintaining good physical and mental health. Studies, including the *Okinawa Centurian Study*, suggest that their extended lifespan is the result of both *genetic and lifestyle factors.*

Genetics and Longevity

- Research shows that the siblings of Okinawa centurions have a much higher likelihood of reaching advanced ages themselves, suggesting a strong genetic component in their ability to resist age-related diseases. Some key genetic traits found in Okinawa include:
    - **Lower inflammation levels**, which reduce the **risk of cardiovascular diseases and autoimmune conditions.**

    - **Efficient metabolism**, helping maintain *a* **healthy weight and prevent obesity** related diseases.

    - **Lower IGF-1** (Insulin-like Growth Factor 1) levels, associated with slower aging and **reduced risk of certain cancers.**

However, genetics alone do not guarantee longevity. Okinawan women's *daily habits, diet, and social connections* play an equally important role *in shaping their health.*

Lower Incidence of Chronic Diseases

Historically, Okinawan women **have significantly lower rates of:**

- **Heart disease and stroke**, due to a **diet low in saturated fats and rich in omega-3 fatty acids** from fish and seaweed.

- **Osteoporosis,** thanks to high consumption of **calcium-rich foods** like tofu and green leafy vegetables.

- Studies suggest that the **lower prevalence** of hormone-related cancers in women like **breast, ovarian and uterine cancers,** might be linked to the high consumption of phytoestrogens, plant-derived compounds with estrogen-like activity, in their diet, particularly from soya-based foods such as miso and tofu.

Their physical activity, whether through **gardening, walking,** or traditional martial arts (*karate and tai chi*), further supports bone health, cardiovascular function, and overall well-being.

Traditional Okinawa Diet: A Model of Longevity

A key aspect of Okinawan health is their plant-based diet, which follows the 80% rule (*Hara Hachi Bu*) – eating until they are justified, not full. Their meal emphasizes:

Core Foods in the Okinawa Diet

- **Sweet potatoes** – A rich source of fiber, vitamins, and antioxidants, replacing rice as the primary carbohydrates.

- **Soy-Based Foods (tofu, miso, natto)** – Providing high quality proteins and phytoestrogens that support hormonal balance.

- **Seaweed** – Packed with minerals like iodine, essential for thyroid health.

- **Bitter Melon** (Goya) – Known for its antidiabetic properties and blood sugar regulation.

- **Turmeric and Green Tea** – Both have powerful anti-inflammatory and antioxidant benefits.

- **Small portions of Fish and Fermented Foods** – Supporting gut health and providing omega-3 fatty acids.

Okinawa- Inspired Meal Plan for Women's Health

- To help integrate *Ikigai-aligned* nutrition into everyday life, here is a sample meal plan inspired by Okinawan dietary principles:

- **Breakfast:** Miso soup with tofu, wakame seaweed, and green onions + steamed sweet potatoes + green tea.

Benefits: High in protein, iodine, and probiotics for gut health.

- **Lunch:** Stir-fried bitter melon with tofu and carrots + brown rice + fermented pickles (tsukemono).

Benefits: Rich in protein, omega-3 fatty acids, iron, calcium and fiber: supports metabolism, hormonal balance, and bone health.

- **Dinner:** Grilled fish (salmon or mackerel) with a side of sauteed spinach and shitake mushrooms + a small serving of natto (fermented soybeans).

Benefits: Heart-healthy omga-3 fatty acids, antioxidants, and slow-digesting carbs.

Snack: A handful of nuts and seeds + a cup of turmeric tea.

This meal plan balances macronutrients and micronutrients while true to the Okinawa diet's longevity principles.

Tofu *is a good source of protein and has high levels of calcium, magnesium, iron, and vitamin B5. It can be a healthy part of most people's diet. It can be more suitable for vegans, vegetarians, and others looking for high protein diet alternative to meat.*

*Along with high protein content, **paneer** is also known to come with high fat content. Every 100 gm of panner contains about 20.8 gm of fat. Tofu, on the other hand contains only 2.7 gm of fat every 100 gm. Due to its low-fat content, tofu is an excellent healthy option for weight loss.*

Japanese sweet potatoes *are incredibly rich in nutrients. This variety is particularly rich in antioxidant and fiber, while regular sweet potato is known for its high vitamins. Again, Japanese sweet potatoes have a lower glycemic index, making them a better option for maintaining stable blood sugar levels.*

Seaweed *is a nutritious food that contains carbohydrates, protein, fiber, magnesium, vitamins and minerals. Seaweed can support health, immunity, promote skin health, and thyroid health because of its iodine content.*

Bitter Melon *is a superfood and one of the healthiest vegetables in the food kingdom. Bitter melon is packed with several key nutrients. It contains iron, magnesium, potassium, vitamin C, vitamin A and much more. A research review* *concluded that bitter melon possesses potent anti-inflammatory and managing inflammation-related properties.*

Green Tea *is a beverage or dietary supplement that may improve mental alertness, relieve digestive symptoms and headaches, and help with weight loss. It's been a popular drink as well as a traditional medicine in Japan and China for thousands of years. It has many health benefits.*

The Changing Landscape: What Can We Learn?

Unfortunately, younger generations in Okinawa are moving away from their traditional diet and adopting more processed foods, refined grains, and sugary beverages, leading to rising rates of obesity, diabetes and heart disease.

However, their longevity secrets can still be applied globally. By adopting elements of the Okinawan way of eating and living, women can support hormonal balance, bone health and disease prevention at every stage of life.

Takeaways for Women's Health

- ✓ Practice the 80% rule (**Hara Hachi Bu**) – Eat mindfully and stop before filling full.

- ✓ Prioritize plant-based foods – Increase vegetables, legumes, and fermented foods.

- ✓ Reduce Processed and Sugary Foods – Limit refined carbs and added sugars.

- ✓ Stay active daily – Engage in walking, gardening, or gentle movement practices like yoga or tai chi.

✓ Foster strong Social Connections – Community and emotional well-being are just as vital as diet.

By integrating such principles, women worldwide can embrace Ikigai-inspired health principles to live longer, healthier and more fulfilling lives.

CHAPTER III: ADOLESCENCE AND THE FOUNDATION OF IKIGAI

"From adolescence to menopause,

a woman's Ikigai evolves, not fades—

each stage offering new ways to thrive,

love, and contribute."

-Anonymous

Adolescence is a period of transformation, especially for girls, as they experience **physical, emotional, and psychological changes**. The Japanese concept of **Ikigai**, meaning "reason for being" or "a life worth living," can provide **purpose, balance, and resilience** during this phase.

First, we will see the physical and emotional changes that occur during adolescence and then how Ikigai can normalize it by applying its principles.

The word adolescence comes from the Latin word adolescere which means "to grow up" or "to mature". It is a unique transitional phase of development that involves rapid physical, cognitive and psychological growth.

World Health Organization (WHO) defines adolescent as someone between the ages 10 and 19 years.

One in every 6 people are aged between 10 and 19 years. Adolescence is the unique stage in life. Physical, emotional and social changes including exposure to poverty, abuse or violence can make adolescents vulnerable to mental health problems.

Mental health conditions are common in adolescent girls, including anxiety, depression, eating disorders and addictive behaviors.

Protecting adolescents from adversity, promoting socio-emotional learning and psychological wellbeing is crucial for their health and wellbeing. Also ensuring access to mental health care is equally important.

According to the World Health Organization (WHO):

- 3.6% of 10 – 14 years old and 4.6% of 15 – 19 years old experience anxiety disorders.

- 1.1% of 10 – 14 years and 2.8% of 15 – 19 years old experience depression.

- ***Adolescent girls are about twice as likely to experience depression as compared to boys.***

The major landmark of puberty for female is **menarche** – the appearance of first menses which usually occurs between the ages 12 and 13 years. The onset of puberty in girls is marked by thelarche – development of breast buds which typically occurs after 8 years of age. Thelarche is followed by adrenarche – appearance of axillary and pubic hairs and finally menarche. We will see here systematically the changes during pubertal development and the challenges the adolescent girls have to face during this phase of life and strategies to tackle it.

Pubertal Physical Changes:

(A) Menarche - The first menstrual period in a life of an adolescent girl.

- **Age at Menarche:** Age at menarche varies significantly among girls and the range of factors contribute to this variation.

Typical Age Range:

- ✓ Average Age around 12.4 years.
- ✓ Range generally between 10 and 16 years.
- ✓ Early menarche before 10 years.
- ✓ Late menarche after 15 years.

- **Factors influencing the age at menarche:**

✓ **Genetics:**

- o Approximately half of the variations in age at menarche are attributed to genetically induced factors.
- o Family history of early or late menarche can be an indicator.

✓ **Nutritional Status:**

- o Adequate healthy nutrition is essential for healthy development and can influence the age at menarche.

- o In Undernourished or Malnourished girls, menarche can be delayed.

✓ **Body Mass Index (BMI):**

- o Girls with higher BMI are associated with earlier menarche.
- o This may be due to increased production of estradiol, a female sex hormone in adipose tissue.

✓ **Socio-economic Factors:**

- o Girls with higher socio-economic background tend to experience menarche earlier than those from lower socio-economic background.
- o This may be due to better nutrition and overall better living conditions.

✓ **Other Factors:**

- o Ethnic Factors: Ethnic and racial differences can influence age at menarche.
- o Geographical location and/or climate can also play a role.
- o Chronic illnesses and exposure to certain drugs can affect the timing of menarche.

Early and or late menarche may be a sign of underlying medical condition and should be discussed with and investigated as per the advice of healthcare provider.

Impact of Menstruation on Mental Health:

- **Physical Changes:**
  - Adolescent girls may feel unprepared for the physical changes associated with menstruation.
  - There may be inadequate access to sanitary pads, inappropriate school/WASH facilities.

- **Emotional Impact:**
  Menarche may trigger feelings of confusion, embarrassment, or even shame due to stigma and lack of adequate education.

Premenstrual Syndrome (PMS):

- **Physical Symptoms:**
  Symptoms like bloating, breast tenderness and fatigue can disrupt daily activities and affect quality of life.

- **Emotional Symptoms:**
  Mood swings, irritability and anxiety are common, impacting relationships and mental wellbeing.

Premenstrual Dysphoric Disorder (PMDD):

- **Severe Emotional Symptoms:**
  PMDD involves more severe emotional symptoms such as severe depression, irritability and mood swings, which significantly impair daily functioning and quality of life.

- **Impact on Mental Health:**
  PMDD can exacerbate existing mental health conditions like depression and anxiety, leading to increased distress and reduced coping abilities.

Dysmenorrhea (Menstrual Cramps):

- **Pain and Discomfort:**
  Dysmenorrhea involves severe menstrual cramps that can interfere with daily activities, causing absenteeism from schools and work places.

- **Psychological Impact:**
  Chronic pain can lead to feelings of frustration, helplessness and even depression, affecting overall mental wellbeing.

Menorrhagia (Heavy Menstrual Bleeding):

- **Physical Consequences:**
  Excessive bleeding can lead to anemia, fatigue and physical discomfort, affecting day-to-day activities.

- **Emotional Strain:**
  Coping with heavy bleeding and its consequences may lead to anxiety, stress and feelings of inadequacy or embarrassment.

Gynecological Strategies to Tackle Challenges:

- **Comprehensive Education:**
  - Provide education about menstruation and menstrual health in schools and communities to empower girls with knowledge and reduce stigma.

  - Offer age-appropriate information about the menstrual cycle, hygiene practices and available resources for managing menstrual health.

- **Access to Healthcare:**
  - If a girl hasn't had her periods by the age 13 and hasn't developed secondary sexual characters (such as development of breast buds, axillary and

pubic hairs), it is recommended to see a healthcare provider especially a qualified gynaecologist to rule out any underlying medical condition.

- o If a girl hasn't had her periods by the age 13, but has well developed secondary sexual characters and is having monthly cyclical pain in abdomen and is having lumpish feel in lower abdomen or pelvic region, it is recommended to visit healthcare provider. It could be a case of cryptomenorrhea (hidden menstruation due to imperforate hymen) which requires treatment.

- o If the girl hasn't had her periods by the age 15 with developed secondary sexual characters but is suffering from chronic health conditions, it is better to visit healthcare provider for further evaluation.

  - ✓ Chronic health conditions such as autoimmune disease like celiac disease, diabetes can delay menarche.
  - ✓ Conditions like hypothyroidism and hyperthyroidism can affect hormonal levels, potentially delaying menarche.
  - ✓ Eating disorders like anorexia nervosa can affect hormonal levels, further delaying menarche.

- o If a girl hasn't had her periods by the age 15, has well developed secondary sexual characters, no chronic health condition or no other complaints;

then her family history needs to be taken into consideration. If a mother or sister started menstruating later than average, it might be normal for the girl to follow a similar pattern.

o Ensure access to healthcare services for menstrual health concerns, including regular check-ups, screening and treatment options for conditions like PMDD, dysmenorrhea and menorrhagia.

o Encourage open communication with healthcare providers to address concerns and seek appropriate management strategies.

Delayed menarche can cause anxiety and emotional distress for the girl and her parents. Visiting a qualified health professional can help address these concerns and provide support.

- **Psychosocial Support:**
  o Create safe places for girls to discuss menstrual health and related concerns, fostering peer support and mutual understanding.

  o Offer counseling services or support groups for girls experiencing emotional distress or mental health challenges associated with menstruation.

- **Self-care Practices:**
  o Encourage girls to practice self-care techniques such as regular exercises, stress management, healthy diet and adequate sleep to alleviate symptoms and improve overall wellbeing.

- o Promote the use of relaxation techniques like medication, yoga or deep breathing exercises to reduce stress and manage emotional symptoms.

- **Policy and Advocacy:**
  - o Advocate for policies that promote menstrual equity, including access to affordable menstrual products, menstrual hygienic facilities and menstrual leave policies in workplaces and schools if needed.

  - o Challenge societal taboos and stigma surrounding menstruation through public awareness campaigns and media representation.

By addressing these challenges systematically through education, access to healthcare, support networks, self-care practices and advocacy efforts, we can better tackle the impact of menarche and menstrual health concerns on adolescent girl's mental health and overall wellbeing.

(B) Development of Secondary Sexual Characters:

- **Thelarche:**

  - This refers to the first noticeable sign of puberty in the form of breast development, typically occurring between the ages 8 and 13.

  - Small firm mounds of tissue form under the nipple known as breast buds.

  - The areola, the pigmented area around the nipple, also enlarges and darkens.

Impact of Breast Development on Mental Health:

  - **Breast Buds:**
    Development of breast buds can lead to feelings of self-consciousness, body image issues and comparisons with peers.

- **Adrenarche:**

  - This refers to the activation of adrenal glands, which produce sex hormones like androgens including testosterone.

  - Adrenarche typically starts around the same time as thelarche, but it can be earlier or later.

  - Androgen plays crucial role in various pubertal changes including:
    - ✓ Growth of axillary and pubic hairs.
    - ✓ Increased oil production in skin leading to acne.
    - ✓ Deepening of voice.

✓ Development of adult body odour.
✓ Maturation of genetalia.

Impact of Adrenarche on Mental Health:

o **Pubic and Axillary Hairs:**
Growing body hair can cause embarrassment especially if it occurs earlier or later than peers, leading to social stigma and insecurity.

o **Acne:**
Hormonal changes during puberty can trigger acne breakouts, affecting self-esteem and confidence, particularly if severe and persistent.

o **Emotional and Psychological Changes:** Mood swings, increased self-awareness and exploration of identity.

(C) Growth Spurt:

o **Increase in Height:**
A rapid increase in height, often accompanied by changes in body proportions. This growth spurt usually begins around ages 9 – 11 years and peaks around ages 12 – 14, but the timings can vary. On an average, girls gain about 8 – 10 inches (20 – 25 cm) in height during this period. The growth plates in long bones, like those in arms and legs, close towards the end of puberty, signalise the end of significant height increase.

o **Increase in Weight:**
Body weight tends to increase during puberty, partly due to increase in muscle mass and body fat. This weight gain is essential for normal development. Girls often experience changes in body composition, redistributing fat to areas like the hips and breasts, leading to a more curvaceous body shape.

o **Body Contour:**
Puberty brings about changes in body contour as fat distribution alters, resulting in a more defined waistline, broader hips and the development of breasts. These changes are influenced by hormonal fluctuations, particularly estrogen, which plays a significant role in shaping the female body during puberty.

o **Genital Organ Changes:**
✓ **Ovaries:** Ovaries change their shape; the elongated shape becomes bulky and oval. The ovarian bulk is due to the follicular enlargement at various stages of development and proliferation of stromal cells.

✓ **The Uterine Body and the Cervix:** The ratio at birth is about 1:2, the ratio becomes 1:1 when menarche occurs. Thereafter the enlargement of the body occurs rapidly, so that the ratio soon becomes 2: 1.

✓ **The Vaginal Changes:** are more pronounced. A few layers of thin epithelium in a girl becomes stratified epithelium of many layers. They are rich in glycogen due to the effect of estrogen. The Doderlein's bacilli appear which convert glycogen into lactic acid. The vaginal ph becomes acidic, ranging between 4 and 5.

It is important to remember that puberty progresses differently in every girl and it's unique for every girl. The timing and sequence of changes can vary. Some girls may experience all these changes simultaneously, while others may have different intervals between them. If the parents have any concerns about pubertal development of their daughter, they should visit a qualified healthcare professional for further advice.

Impact of Growth Spurt on Mental Health:

- Rapid physical growth can lead to feelings of clumsiness, discomfort and dissatisfaction with one's changing body shape.

- Height disparities with peers can contribute to feelings of self-consciousness, inadequacy or being different.

- **Body Image Concerns:**
  Changes in physical appearance may lead to negative body image perceptions, low self-esteem and increased vulnerability to eating disorders.

- **Social Pressure:**
Peer comparisons and societal beauty standards can exacerbate feelings of insecurity, isolation and fear of rejection.

- **Emotional Distress:**
Coping with physical changes and societal expectations may lead to stress, anxiety and depression, affecting overall mental wellbeing.

- **Media Representation:**
  o The media often portrays unrealistic beauty standards, promoting thinness and flawless appearance as the ideal.

  o Images of airbrushed models and celebrities can distort perceptions of normal body shapes and sizes.

  o Constant exposure to edited photos and influenced culture can lead to feelings of inadequacy and self-comparison.

- **Peer Comparison:**
  o Adolescents frequently compare themselves to their peers, striving to meet societal beauty ideal.

  o Peer groups may reinforce certain body standards through comments, jokes or social media interactions.

- **Family Influence:**
  o Family attitudes and behaviors regarding body image can shape adolescent's perception of herself.

(D) How Ikegai Can Help Adolescent Girls Navigate Growth, Identity, Body Image Emotions and Self-worth?

Ikigai consists of **four key elements**:

1. **What you love (Passion)**
2. **What you are good at (Talent)**
3. **What the world needs (Purpose)**
4. **What can sustain you (Potential Growth)**

By aligning these elements, adolescent girls can **cope with changes, build self-confidence, and develop a positive self-image**.

How Ikigai Helps in Navigating Physical Changes

1. Coping with Body Image Issues

- Many girls feel **self-conscious** about weight gain, height changes, or acne.
- **Ikigai helps them focus on their strengths** beyond appearance—talents, hobbies, and skills—fostering self-worth.
- Practicing **gratitude for a healthy body** can help develop body positivity.

✓ **Example:** Engaging in activities like **dance, sports, or yoga** can help girls appreciate their bodies' strength rather than just appearance.

2. Managing Emotional Swings and Stress

- Hormonal fluctuations lead to **mood swings, anxiety, and self-doubt**.
- Ikigai encourages **self-reflection** and finding a **personal anchor**, such as journaling, meditation, or art to process emotions.

- A sense of purpose helps them **redirect stress into creative or meaningful activities**.

✓ **Example:** If a girl finds joy in **writing or painting**, she can channel emotional ups and downs into a creative outlet, helping with emotional regulation.

3. Overcoming Peer Pressure and Comparison

- Girls often compare themselves to others, leading to **low self-esteem**.
- Ikigai encourages them to **identify their unique strengths and passions** instead of following societal or peer-imposed standards.
- Developing **a strong sense of purpose** makes them less likely to seek validation from social media or peer groups.

✓ **Example:** If a girl realizes she loves **helping animals**, she can volunteer at a shelter, finding fulfillment beyond external validation.

4. Building Resilience and Confidence

- Puberty brings **challenges like menstrual discomfort, acne, and fatigue**.
- Instead of feeling ashamed, Ikigai helps them **embrace these changes as part of growth**.
- It encourages them to **adopt healthy habits**, such as nutrition, exercise, and self-care, to respect their bodies.

✓ **Example:** A girl passionate about **fitness or well-being** might start a healthy lifestyle, focusing on balanced nutrition rather than fad diets.

5. Strengthening Social and Family Bonds

- Adolescence often brings **conflicts with parents and misunderstandings with friends**.
- Ikigai promotes **healthy communication, gratitude, and emotional intelligence**, helping girls build stronger relationships.
- It guides them to **surround themselves with supportive, like-minded individuals** who uplift them.

✓ **Example:** If a girl values **community service**, she can join a group that aligns with her interests, fostering meaningful friendships.

Applying Ikigai in Daily Life for Adolescent Girls

1. **Self-Discovery Journaling** – Write about what makes them happy and gives them purpose.

2. **Mindfulness & Gratitude** – Appreciate the journey of growing up instead of fearing changes.

3. **Engaging in Meaningful Activities** – Sports, art, music, volunteering—anything that sparks joy.

4. **Surrounding Themselves with Positive Influences** – Friends and mentors who support growth.

5. **Embracing Self-Acceptance** – Understanding that everyone's journey is unique and beautiful.

In summary, by integrating Ikigai into their daily lives, adolescent girls can navigate physical and emotional changes with confidence, purpose, and resilience. It helps them embrace their uniqueness, overcome insecurities, and find joy in their evolving selves.

(E) The Risk-taking behaviours in Adolescent Girls:

The risk-taking behaviors in Adolescent Girls related to substance abuse, self-harm and risky sexual behavior and resources for seeking help:

Substance Abuse:

- Experimentation with drugs, smoking or alcohol as a means of coping with stress, peer pressure or curiosity.

- Consequences may include addiction, impaired cognitive function, physical health problems, academic or legal issues and strained relationships with family and peers.

- **Resources for seeking help include:**
  - School counselors or nurses who can provide support and guidance.

  - Substance abuse hotlines or helplines or confidential assistance.

  - Rehabilitation centers or outpatient programs specializing in substance abuse treatment.

Self-harm:

- Engaging in self-harm behaviors such as cutting, burning or hitting oneself as a way to cope with emotional pain or distress.

- Consequences may include physical injury, scarring, infection, worsening mental health symptoms and potential escalation of self-harm behaviors.

- **Resources for seeking help include:**
  - Mental health professionals such as therapists, counselors or psychiatrists who can provide therapy and support.

  - Crisis hotlines or helplines staffed by trained professionals who can offer immediate assistance and referral to appropriate services.

  - Support groups or online communities for individuals struggling with self-harm to connect with others and share experiences.

Risky Sexual Behavior:

- Engaging in unprotected sex, multiple sexual partners or sexual activity under the influence of drugs or alcohol.

- Consequences may include unintended pregnancy, sexually transmitted infections (STIs), emotional trauma, relationship conflicts and social stigma.

- **Resources for seeking help include:**
  - Sexual help clinics or Planned Parenthood Centers for confidential STIs testing, contraception and reproductive health services.

  - School counselors or nurses who can provide education on safe sex practices and referrals to appropriate resources.

  - Mental health professionals who specialize in sexual health and relationships and who can offer support and guidance in navigating sexual decision-making.

In each case it is crucial for adolescent girls to understand the potential consequences of these risk-taking behaviors and to seek help from trusted adults or professional resources when needed. Engaging open communication and reducing stigma surrounding these issues can help adolescents feel more comfortable seeking support and accessing necessary resources for their wellbeing.

(F) How Ikigai Helps Adolescent Girls Overcome Challenges Related to Risk-Taking Behaviors

Adolescence is a time of **exploration, independence, and curiosity**, but it is also a period where **risk-taking behaviors**—such as impulsive decisions, peer pressure, and experimentation—can become a challenge. The **Ikigai framework** provides adolescent girls with a **sense of direction, purpose, and self-awareness**, helping them make healthier choices.

Ikigai consists of **four key elements,** already discussed.

By **identifying their Ikigai**, girls can develop **self-discipline, confidence, and inner strength** to **resist negative influences** and focus on meaningful growth.

Common Risk-Taking Behaviors in Adolescent Girls

- Peer pressure to engage in smoking, drinking, or substance use.

- Reckless social media behavior (oversharing, online bullying, seeking validation).

- Unprotected or early sexual activity due to lack of awareness.

- Breaking rules and engaging in thrill-seeking activities (vandalism, shoplifting, skipping school, etc.)

- Self-harm, eating disorders, or extreme dieting due to body image issues.

Why do these behaviors occur?

- **Brain development:** The prefrontal cortex (responsible for decision-making) is still developing, leading to **impulsivity**.

- **Social belonging:** The need for approval can push girls toward **risky behaviors** to fit in.

- **Emotional turbulence:** Mood swings, low self-esteem, or identity struggles may lead to **reckless choices**.

How Ikigai Helps Reduce Risk-Taking Behaviors

Ikigai helps **redirect energy toward positive, fulfilling activities**, reducing the likelihood of engaging in harmful behaviors.

1. Strengthens Self-Identity & Reduces Peer Pressure

- Adolescent girls who have **a clear sense of purpose (Ikigai)** are less likely to **give in to negative peer influence**.

- They build **self-confidence** and make choices based on their personal values, rather than **seeking validation from friends or social media**.

✓ **Example:** If a girl identifies her Ikigai as **"helping animals"**, she may spend time volunteering at an animal shelter rather than engaging in risky behavior for social acceptance.

2. Helps Channel Curiosity into Positive Risk-Taking

- Not all risks are bad! Ikigai encourages **constructive risk-taking**, such as:
    - o Exploring a **new sport or hobby**

    - o Taking leadership roles in school

    - o Starting a **social initiative**

- Instead of engaging in **dangerous behaviors**, girls feel excitement in **pushing their limits in safe and meaningful ways**.

✓ **Example:** A girl who loves **public speaking** might push herself to **join a debate competition** rather than seeking thrills through unsafe activities.

3. Develops Self-Control & Decision-Making Skills

- Knowing **what truly matters** helps girls think before making impulsive decisions.

- Ikigai encourages **goal-setting and future thinking**, making them pause before taking unnecessary risks.

✓ **Example:** A girl passionate about **becoming a doctor** will be **less likely to engage in substance abuse** because she understands its long-term impact on her future.

4. Provides Emotional Stability & Reduces Self-Destructive Behavior

Many risk-taking behaviors stem from **emotional pain, low self-esteem, or stress**.

- Ikigai helps girls find **healthy coping mechanisms** like:

- o **Journaling** to process emotions.

  - o **Exercise or meditation** for stress relief.

  - o **Creative arts (painting, music, writing)** to channel inner struggles.

✓ **Example:** A girl feeling insecure about her body may turn to **fitness, dance, or yoga** instead of unhealthy dieting or self-harm.

5. Encourages Meaningful Social Connections

- Ikigai **helps girls find like-minded friends** who support their growth instead of influencing negative behavior.

- When surrounded by **positive role models**, they are less likely to **seek approval from toxic friendships**.

✓ **Example:** A girl passionate about **the environment** may join an **eco-club**, making friends who share similar values rather than those who pressure her into unhealthy habits.

Practical Ways to Apply Ikigai for Risk Management

1. **Self-Discovery Activities:** Encourage girls to write down **what excites them, what they're good at, and what they want to contribute to the world**.

2. **Engage in Skill-Building Activities:** Help them explore **sports, arts, music, leadership roles, community work, or learning new skills**.

3. **Mindfulness & Reflection:** Teach them **meditation, gratitude practices, or vision boards** to align with their Ikigai.

4. **Encourage Safe Exploration:** Let them **try new things** in a controlled and positive environment.

In summary, Ikigai helps adolescent girls gain a sense of purpose, self-confidence, and emotional resilience—reducing the tendency to engage in harmful risk-taking behaviors. By channeling their energy into fulfilling activities, they make wiser choices and build a future based on passion and purpose.

(G) Guided Ikigai Worksheet Designed to Help Adolescent Girls

Here is a **Guided Ikigai Worksheet** designed to help **adolescent girls explore their purpose, align their passions, and reduce risky behaviors**. It includes reflection questions, activities, and goal-setting exercises to **redirect energy toward positive and meaningful pursuits**.

Discover your purpose, overcome challenges, and make better choices through Ikigai.

Step 1: Self-Reflection – Who Are You?

→ **Think about yourself. Answer the following questions honestly.**

- What are **three things** that make you excited or happy every day?
  Example: Drawing, listening to music, helping friends.
- What are some **things you do naturally well** without much effort?
  Example: Writing, playing sports, comforting others.
- What activities make you **lose track of time** because you enjoy them so much?
  Example: Reading, dancing, solving puzzles
- When someone asks you, "What do you want to do in the future?" what's your answer?
  Example: Become a doctor, travel the world, teach children.

Step 2: Understanding Your Strengths – What Are You Good At?

→ **List some of your skills and talents that you can improve on.**

- I am good at _______________________
- My friends/family say I am good at _______________________
- I feel confident when I _______________________

Step 3: Finding Your Passion – What Do You Love?

→ **Write down what excites you the most.**

- If I could spend a whole day doing one thing, it would be _______________________
- I feel the happiest when I am _______________________
- A topic I can talk about for hours without getting bored is _______________________

Step 4: Identifying Your Purpose – What Can You Contribute to the World?

→ **How do you want to make a difference in the world or help others?**

- I feel most useful when I _______________________
- I wish I could help others by _______________________
- If I could solve one problem in the world, it would be _______________________

Step 5: Aligning Your Ikigai – Your Path to a Meaningful Life

→ **Bring everything together!**

- My **Ikigai** (Reason for Being) is:
  I love _______________________
- I am good at _______________________
- The world needs _______________________
- I can grow in this area by _______________________

Step 6: Overcoming Risky Behaviors with Ikigai

→ **Think about challenges you face and how Ikigai can help.**

- One negative behavior or habit I want to avoid: _____
- A healthy activity I will do instead: _____________
- A person I can talk to for support: _____________
- A goal I will set for the next month: ___________

Example:

- **I want to avoid:** Skipping school because of peer pressure.
- **Instead, I will:** Join a book club that helps me grow.
- **I will talk to:** My best friend or teacher when I feel lost.
- **My goal will be:** Read one new book every month and share my thoughts.

Step 7: Daily Ikigai Practice – Action Plan

→ **Turn your Ikigai into action!**

Daily Habit Tracker

- Today, I will spend at least **30 minutes** on an activity I love.
- I will surround myself with **positive people** who support me.
- I will avoid **negative influences** by staying focused on my goals.

This worksheet guides adolescent girls' step by step in finding their purpose, reducing peer pressure, making better choices, and staying motivated.

CHAPTER IV: MOTHERHOOD AND FOUNDATION OF IKIGAI

"To invest in women's health

is to invest in the future of humanity".

-Anonymous

Motherhood is a transformative journey that brings joy, challenges and profound changes to a woman's life. Amid the joyous moment and new beginning, it is essential to acknowledge the less discussed aspects of motherhood, particularly those related to mental health.

The transition to motherhood is marked by hormonal fluctuations, sleep deprivation and adjustment to a new role, potentially impacting a women's mental wellbeing.

The journey through motherhood, especially when complicated by delayed marriages due to carrier opportunities, infertility, abortions or bad obstetric history and further exacerbated by the pursuit of IVF and its financial implications; can significantly impact a woman's mental health.

The transition from adulthood to motherhood is a potentially vulnerable time for some women's mental health and approximately 9 – 21% of women experience depression and anxiety at this time. Many more experience subclinical symptoms of depression and/or anxiety, stress, low esteem and loss of confidence.

Postpartum mental disorders, including postpartum depression, anxiety disorders and even rare but severe cases of postpartum psychosis; can throw a shadow over this joyous moment of being mother.

In reproductive years, impact on women's mental health can be addressed in different stages including selecting a perfect life partner, preparing and navigating the journey of motherhood, postpartum mental health, balancing career, family and parental responsibilities.

(A) Impact on Mental Health of a Woman while Navigating through Motherhood:

Navigating through motherhood can pose significant challenges to a woman's mental health, especially when facing delays in conceiving due to carrier opportunities, infertility, repeated abortions and/or a bad obstetric history leading to pursuit of IVF (In-Vitro-Fertilization) and the associated financial burden.

Delay in Conceiving Due to Career Opportunities:

The best age to marry a girl, or anyone for that matter is a highly individual and subjective matter that can vary depending on personal circumstances, cultural norms and individual preferences. There is no **"one size fits-all answer"** to this question as people mature and develop at different rates, have different life goals and face different challenges.

It is important to note that marriage is a significant life decision that should not be rushed into. Factors such as emotional maturity, financial stability, readiness for commitment, compatibility with the partner and personal goals should all be taken into consideration when deciding for right time for marriage.

Dr. Fisher believes that marriages that take place when the couple is in their late 20s and mid 30s are most successful. "By the time we are getting to late 20s, we have a clear sense of who we are and what we want out of life," he explains.

But this trend is changing in recent years with people choosing to marry later in life for various reasons such as pursuing education, personal goals and personal development and may land in:

- Feelings of frustration, anxiety or guilt about postponing motherhood for pursuing education, carrier later in life.

- There can be pressure from societal expectations or family members to prioritize either carrier or motherhood.

Infertility:

Pregnancy and child-bearing are key life events and studies have shown the happiness of mother, the couple as a whole before, during and after childbirth.

Some believe that pregnancy can make you aware of the world around you and that preparing for the baby can make you feel more secure and confident. Family members often treat you well when they hear you are pregnant.

Inability to conceive naturally can cause feelings of shame, guilt and low self-esteem. These negative feelings may lead varying degrees of depression, anxiety, distress and a poor quality of life.

Studies have shown that infertile couples experience significant anxiety and emotional distress, when fertility treatment proves to be unsuccessful, for instance, women and couples can experience deep feelings of grief and loss.

Infertility can lead to:

- Emotional distress including feelings of inadequacy, sadness or despair.

- Strain on relationships, as fertility can cause tension between partners.

- Social isolation such as interaction with friends or family members without children may become difficult.

- Loss of self-esteem and identity tied to traditional notions of womanhood or motherhood.

Repeated Abortions can lead to:

- Psychological trauma, including guilt, shame or grief.

- Fear of future pregnancies and anxieties about potential complications.

- Impact on mental wellbeing, potentially leading to depression or anxiety disorders.

Bad Obstetric History can lead to:

- PTSD (Post-Traumatic Stress Disorder) symptoms due to traumatic childbirth experiences.

- Anxiety and fear surrounding subsequent pregnancies or childbirth.

- Grief and mourning for lost pregnancies or children.

In-Vitro Fertilization (IVF) and Financial Burden can lead to:

- Stress and anxiety related to the IVF process, including hormonal treatments, injections and medical procedures.

- Financial strain from the high costs of IVF, leading to worries about financial instability.

- Feelings of guilt or pressure to justify the financial investment, especially when unsuccessful even with IVF.

- Impact on overall wellbeing, as financial stressors can exacerbate existing mental health issues.

(B) How to Tackle the Impact on Mental Health for a Woman Navigating through Motherhood.

Seeking Professional Support:

- Encourage women to seek support from mental health professionals such as therapists or counselors, who specialize in fertility issues and maternal mental health.

- Provide information about support groups or online communities where women can connect with others who have experienced similar challenges.

Open Communication:

- Encourage open communication between partners to share feelings, concerns and expectations about the journey to parenthood.

- Facilitate discussions about coping strategies, including how to manage stress and anxiety together.

Education and Information:

- Offer education about fertility, reproductive health and the IVF process to empower the women with knowledge and understanding.

- Provide resources and information about potential risks, challenges and success rates associated with IVF treatment.

Emotional Support:

- Offer emotional support to address feelings of grief, loss or disappointment related to delayed conception and bad obstetric history.

- Validate the women's emotions and provide a safe space for her to express her feelings without judgement.

Self-Care Practices:

- Encourage self-care practices such as mindfulness, relaxation techniques, exercise and hobbies to help manage stress and promote overall wellbeing.

- Emphasize the importance of self-compassion and self-kindness throughout the journey.

Building a Support Network:

- Encourage the woman to build a strong support network of friends, family and healthcare professionals who can offer practical and emotional support.

- Provide resources for connecting with other women who have experienced similar challenges through support groups or online forums.

Addressing Financial Concerns:

- Offer guidance on financial planning and resources for managing the financial burden of IVF treatment, such as exploring insurance coverage, grants or financial assistance programs.

- Help women develop a budget and explore alternative options for financing treatment of infertility, if needed.

Regular Check-ups and Monitoring:

- Schedule regular check-ups with healthcare providers to monitor emotional wellbeing, provides updates on treatment progress and address any concerns or questions.

- Monitor for signs of depression, anxiety or other mental health issues and provide appropriate interventions or referrals as needed.

In summary, by following these approaches, women can successfully navigate through motherhood or even through infertility, and if no success in IVF treatment, then by going for adoption.

(C) Ikigai as a Guide to Navigating Reproductive Health and Motherhood

Reproductive health and motherhood bring immense joy, but they also come with physical, emotional, and societal challenges. From menstrual health to pregnancy, childbirth and postpartum recovery, women often face complex transitions that can impact their well-being. Through the lens of *Ikigai*, women can cultivate resilience, purpose, and balance, transforming these experiences into opportunities for growth and fulfillment.

1. **Emotional and Psychological Resilience**
   - **Finding Purpose Amidst Challenges:** Where dealing with fertility struggles, hormonal imbalances, or postpartum depression, a strong sense of *Ikigai* helps women anchor themselves in meaning and hope.

   - **Emotional Stability:** By aligning with their passions and values, women can navigate mood swings, anxiety, and self-doubt with greater confidence and inner peace.

   - ***Example:***
     Ankita, a 39 years-old marketing professional, struggled for infertility for years. The emotional toll left her feeling lost, but she found strength in her Ikigai-mentoring young professionals. She adopted a girl child and started a blog to support women facing similar challenges, which not only helped her cope but also provided a sense of purpose beyond her struggle.

Lesson:

Even in difficult reproductive health experiences, aligning with one's Ikigai – be it through career, passion, or community service – helps maintain emotional balance and mental well-being.

2. **Prioritizing Physical Well-being**
   - **Holistic Self-Care:** Women often neglect their health while caring for others. *Ikigai* promotes balance, ensuring they prioritize proper nutrition, exercise, and rest.

   - **Healing and Recovery:** From menstrual disorders to pregnancy complications, understanding one's purpose can enhance emotional strength, which positively impacts physical healing and resilience.

   - *Example:*
   Nita, a 29 years-old teacher, experienced severe postpartum depression after her first child. She had always loved yoga but abandoned self-care after giving birth. Her friend reminded her how mindfulness had once brought her joy. Slowly, she reintegrated yoga into her routine, which significantly improved her emotional and physical recovery.

   Lesson:
   Women often deprioritize their well-being, but *Ikigai* encourages self-care as an essential part of a fulfilled life. By reconnecting with activities that bring joy, women can regain strength and vitality.

3. **Harmonizing Career and Motherhood**
   - **Work-Life Integration:** Many women grabble with societal expectations of balancing careers and motherhood. *Ikigai* empowers them to define success on their own terms, ensuring fulfillment in both roles.

   - **Guilt-Free Decision-Making:** Women who embrace their *Ikigai* can confidently make choices – where to pause their careers, pursue entrepreneurship, or continue working – without external pressures dictating their path.

   - *Example:*
   Priya, a software engineer, faced immense guilt returning to work after maternity leave. She loved coding but felt pressured by family to quit her job. After reflecting on her *Ikigai*, she realized her passion for solving problems and mentoring young female engineers was a core part of her identity. She negotiated a flexible work arrangement, allowing her to nurture both her career and family.

   Lesson:
   Ikegai helps women define success on their own terms rather than feeling trapped by societal expectations. A fulfilling life isn't about choosing between career and motherhood – it's about integrating both in a way that aligns with personal purpose.

4. **Strengthening Relationships and Support System**
   - **Building Meaningful Connections:** *Ikigai* fosters deep relationships with partners, family, and communities, providing women with

emotional and practical support needed during motherhood and reproductive health journeys.

- **Raising Emotionally Healthy Children:** A mother aligned with her *Ikigai* nurtures a positive, emotionally stable environment, benefitting her child's psychological and social well-being.

- *Example:*
Namita, a 37-year-old single mother, felt overwhelmed raising her twins alone. She found her *Ikigai* in community service and joined a support group for single mothers, making motherhood more manageable and fulfilling.

- *Lesson:*
Building meaningful relationships is a key component of *Ikigai*. A strong support system enhances emotional resilience and eases the burdens of motherhood and reproductive health struggles.

5. **Empowerment and Self-Identity:**
   - **Beyond the Role of a mother:** Many women struggle with identity loss after childbirth. Ikigai helps them recollect with their passions and personal aspirations while embracing motherhood.

   - **Strengthening Self-Worth:** Understanding their intrinsic value beyond societal expectation enables women to approach reproductive health and motherhood with confidence and purpose.

- *Example:*
  Pravina, a 41-years-old artist, felt she has lost her identity after becoming a mother of two. She has put her painting career on hold for a decade. When her youngest kid started school, she revisited her love of art, taking small steps like painting at home and eventually showcasing her work at local exhibitions. She realized that embracing her creative passion made her a more fulfilled mother.

Lesson: Motherhood is a significant role, but it doesn't have to replace personal identity. *Ikigai* helps women reconnect with their passions, proving that self-fulfillment enhances – not detracts from – family life.

In summary, through the lens of Ikigai, reproductive health and motherhood become more than biological or societal experiences – they transform into deeply personal journeys of meaning, balance, and joy. By aligning with their true purpose, women can navigate challenges with resilience, prioritize self-care, balance career and family, build strong support systems, and maintain a thriving self-identity.

(D) Guided Ikigai Worksheet for Motherhood & the Reproductive Phase

Discovering Purpose, Balance, and Joy in Motherhood

Instructions:
This worksheet is designed to help you reflect on your life as a mother and an individual. Take your time to answer each section thoughtfully.

1. What You Love (Passion)

These are the things that bring you joy, fulfillment, and energy.

- What aspects of motherhood make you truly happy?
  Example: Watching my child grow, bedtime stories, preparing healthy meals, etc.

- What activities make you feel most alive and connected to yourself?
  Example: Writing, gardening, dancing, painting, etc.

- What did you enjoy before becoming a mother that still excites you?
  Example: Reading, traveling, learning new skills, etc.

2. What You Are Good At (Vocation)

Your natural strengths, skills, and talents.

- What skills have you developed as a mother?
  Example: Multitasking, patience, emotional intelligence, problem-solving, etc.

- What are your unique talents outside of motherhood?
  Example: Teaching, writing, cooking, designing, leadership, etc.

- What do people compliment you on?
  Example: Being a good listener, creative ideas, organizing events, etc.

3. What the World (Your Family & Community) Needs (Mission)

Where you can make a difference.

- How do you support and inspire your family?
  Example: By creating a loving home, teaching good values, providing emotional support.

- How can you contribute to your community while being a mother?
  Example: Volunteering at a school, supporting other moms, starting a blog or YouTube channel.

- What message or lesson do you want to pass on to your children?
  Example: Kindness, resilience, self-love, discipline, pursuing dreams, etc.

4. What You Can Be Paid For (Profession)

Balancing career, financial independence, and personal fulfillment.

- How can you turn your skills into a profession or side income?
  Example: Teaching online, blogging, consulting, freelancing, crafting, coaching, etc.

- Are there career opportunities that align with motherhood and your strengths?
  Example: Flexible remote work, starting a small business, content creation, etc.

- How can you manage time effectively between work and family?
  Example: Setting boundaries, prioritizing, outsourcing certain tasks.

Bringing It All Together: Your Ikigai Statement

Write a short paragraph about how you can integrate these four elements (passion, vocation, mission, and profession) into a fulfilling life.

Example:

"I love nurturing and guiding my children while also inspiring other mothers through writing and speaking. My ability to teach and share experiences allows me to create valuable content for moms who seek balance and fulfillment. The world needs strong, happy mothers, and I can contribute by supporting other women through my blog and coaching. I can also turn my passion into a sustainable career by offering online parenting workshops and self-care programs. Through this, I create a life where I feel purposeful, balanced, and financially independent."

Reflection Questions

1. How does this exercise help you redefine your identity beyond motherhood?

2. What is one small action you can take today to align with your Ikigai?

3. What challenges might hold you back, and how can you overcome them?

4. How can you practice self-care and prioritize yourself while being a mother?

CHAPTER V: MENOPAUSE AND REDISCOVERING IKIGAI

"Menopause isn't an end;

it's a new beginning—

an opportunity to redefine your Ikigai

and live with renewed vitality and wisdom."

-Anonymous

(A) Understanding Menopause and Its Short-Term and Long-Term Effects on the Body and Mind

Menopause is a significant phase in a woman's life, marking the end of her reproductive years. It is defined as the cessation of menstruation for 12 consecutive months and typically occurs between the ages of 45 and 55. This transition is driven by a decline in estrogen and progesterone levels, leading to a variety of physiological and psychological changes. Understanding the short-term and long-term effects of menopause on the body and mind is crucial for women to navigate this phase with resilience and a renewed sense of purpose, or ***Ikigai.***

Short-Term Effects of Menopause

- **Vasomotor Symptoms (Hot Flashes & Night Sweats)**
  - o Sudden feelings of heat, flushing, and sweating, often disrupting sleep.

- o Can lead to irritability and fatigue due to poor rest.

- **Menstrual Irregularities**
  - o Periods become erratic before stopping completely.

  - o Heavy or scanty bleeding may occur, sometimes leading to anemia.

- **Mood Swings & Emotional Changes**
  - o Increased irritability, anxiety, or depressive symptoms due to hormonal fluctuations.

  - o Emotional sensitivity and decreased stress tolerance.

- **Sleep Disturbances (Insomnia)**
  - o Difficulty falling or staying asleep.

  - o Night sweats contribute to poor sleep quality, leading to daytime fatigue.

- **Cognitive Fog & Memory Issues**
  - o Difficulty concentrating and forgetfulness.

  - o Temporary cognitive decline often referred to as "brain fog."

- **Weight Gain & Metabolic Changes**
  - o Slower metabolism leading to weight gain, especially around the abdomen.

  - o Increased insulin resistance raising the risk of type 2 diabetes.

- **Vaginal Dryness & Sexual Discomfort**
  - o Reduced estrogen causes thinning of vaginal tissues, leading to dryness, itching, and pain during intercourse.

  - o Decreased libido or changes in sexual satisfaction.

- **Skin & Hair Changes**
  - o Loss of collagen results in dry, thinning skin and increased wrinkles.

  - o Hair thinning or loss due to hormonal imbalance.

- **Joint & Muscle Aches**
  - o Increased stiffness and pain in joints and muscles due to declining estrogen's protective effect on inflammation.

Long-Term Effects of Menopause

- **Osteoporosis & Bone Loss**
  - o Estrogen deficiency accelerates bone resorption, leading to decreased bone density and increased fracture risk (osteoporosis).

  - o Higher chances of hip, spine, and wrist fractures.

- **Cardiovascular Disease (CVD) Risk**
  - o Estrogen has a protective effect on heart health, and its decline increases the risk of hypertension, high cholesterol, and heart attacks.

  - o Increased arterial stiffness and risk of atherosclerosis.

- **Cognitive Decline & Dementia Risk**
  - Higher risk of Alzheimer's and other neurodegenerative diseases due to reduced estrogen's neuroprotective role.

  - Increased prevalence of mood disorders such as depression and anxiety.

- **Urinary Incontinence & Pelvic Floor Weakness**
  - Weakening of pelvic muscles leading to stress urinary incontinence and increased susceptibility to urinary tract infections (UTIs).

- **Changes in Body Composition & Metabolic Syndrome**
  - Increased abdominal fat accumulation.

  - Greater risk of metabolic syndrome, leading to diabetes and hypertension.

- **Declining Muscle Mass & Strength (Sarcopenia)**
  - Progressive muscle loss affects mobility, balance, and physical strength.

  - Reduced physical activity can worsen frailty.

- **Vision & Hearing Changes**
  - Increased risk of dry eyes and cataracts.

  - Some women may experience hearing loss due to estrogen decline.

- **Emotional & Social Impact**
  - Feelings of loss of youthfulness, confidence, or attractiveness.

  - Increased loneliness or emotional disconnect if not addressed through social and personal engagement.

(B) Gynecological Advice: Managing Symptoms, Hormone Therapy, and Emotional Well-being

Navigating menopause requires a comprehensive approach that includes managing physical symptoms, exploring hormone therapy options, and ensuring emotional well-being. Gynecologists play a crucial role in guiding women through this transition, helping them make informed choices to maintain their quality of life.

1. Managing Symptoms Naturally and Medically

Menopausal symptoms can range from mild to severe, affecting daily life. A combination of lifestyle modifications, medical treatments, and alternative therapies can help ease the transition.

Lifestyle Changes for Symptom Relief

- **Dietary Adjustments:**
    - Consume calcium and vitamin D-rich foods to support bone health.

    - Incorporate phytoestrogens (soy, flaxseeds, legumes) to naturally balance hormones.

    - Reduce caffeine, alcohol, and spicy foods to minimize hot flashes.

    - Maintain a balanced diet rich in lean protein, whole grains, and healthy fats.

- **Regular Exercise:**
    - Strength training and weight-bearing exercises prevent osteoporosis and maintain muscle mass.

    - Yoga and Pilates improve flexibility and reduce stress.

- o Cardiovascular exercises like walking and swimming support heart health.

- **Hydration and Skincare:**
  - o Drink plenty of water to combat dryness and keep skin hydrated.

  - o Use gentle moisturizers and sun protection to maintain skin elasticity.

- **Pelvic Floor Strengthening:**
  - o Kegel exercises help prevent urinary incontinence and support vaginal health.

  - o Regular pelvic floor therapy can be beneficial for postmenopausal women.

- **Sleep Hygiene:**
  - o Maintain a consistent sleep schedule.

  - o Use cooling blankets and keep the bedroom temperature low to prevent night sweats.

  - o Avoid screen time before bed and practice relaxation techniques like meditation.

Medical Management for Severe Symptoms

If lifestyle changes are not sufficient, medical interventions may be necessary.

- **Non-Hormonal Medications:**
  - o **Antidepressants (SSRIs/SNRIs):** Can help with mood swings, hot flashes, and anxiety.

  - o **Gabapentin & Clonidine:** Effective for hot flashes and sleep disturbances.

o **Ospemifene:** Helps with vaginal dryness and painful intercourse.

- **Vaginal Moisturizers & Lubricants:**
  o Over-the-counter vaginal moisturizers and lubricants improve comfort during intercourse.

  o Prescribing vaginal estrogen (cream, tablet, or ring) can restore vaginal health.

2. Hormone Therapy (HT): Benefits, Risks, and Guidelines

Hormone Therapy (HT), also known as Menopausal Hormone Therapy (MHT), is one of the most effective treatments for managing menopausal symptoms. However, it must be carefully tailored to each woman's health profile.

Types of Hormone Therapy

- **Estrogen Therapy (ET):**
  o Recommended for women who have had a hysterectomy.

  o Available in pills, patches, gels, creams, and vaginal forms.

  o Helps with hot flashes, vaginal dryness, and osteoporosis prevention.

- **Combined Estrogen-Progestin Therapy (EPT):**
  o Given to women with an intact uterus to prevent endometrial hyperplasia.

  o Reduces menopausal symptoms while protecting the uterus from estrogen's effects.

(Details about MHT can be read from my book "Demystifying Menopause Hormone Therapy)

Benefits of Hormone Therapy

- Reduces hot flashes and night sweats.

- Prevents bone loss and fractures.

- Improves vaginal health and reduces discomfort.

- May reduce the risk of colorectal cancer.

- Enhances quality of life and energy levels.

Risks and Considerations

- Slight increase in risk of breast cancer (especially with long-term use of EPT).

- Potential risk of blood clots, stroke, and heart disease in certain women.

- Not recommended for women with a history of breast cancer, blood clots, or severe liver disease.

Who Should Consider HT?

Target population for initiation of therapy is within 10 years of menopause and below 60 years of age. MHT initiated early in symptomatic healthy women is always beneficial and safe.

Risk calculations are applied strictly.

- Taking detailed history.

- Physical examination including breast and pelvis.

- Basic mandatory investigations.

- Special added investigations for some women, if indicated as per history.

- Using "Risk Assessment Tools" for breast cancer and cardiovascular disease.

- Using right MHT, route and duration of therapy.

Alternative Options for Women Who Cannot Take HT

- **Selective Estrogen Receptor Modulators (SERMs)** like Raloxifene for bone health.

- **Tibolone**, a synthetic hormone alternative used in some countries.

- **Herbal and Complementary Therapies** (though evidence is mixed).

3. Emotional Well-being and Mental Health Support

Menopause is not just a physical transformation but also an emotional and psychological shift. Many women experience mood swings, depression, and a loss of self-identity during this stage. Prioritizing mental well-being is crucial for overall health.

Managing Emotional Changes

- **Recognizing Emotional Symptoms**
  o Increased anxiety or irritability.

  o Feelings of sadness or lack of motivation.

  o Difficulty concentrating and memory lapses.

Therapeutic Approaches

- **Cognitive Behavioral Therapy (CBT):** Effective for managing anxiety and mood swings.

- **Mindfulness & Meditation:** Helps in reducing stress and promoting emotional balance.

- **Journaling & Self-Reflection:** Encourages self-awareness and emotional release.

Social Support & Relationships

- Maintain strong relationships with family and friends.

- Join support groups or online communities for menopausal women.

- Communicate openly with partners about changes in intimacy and emotions.

Reconnecting with Purpose and Ikigai

- Engage in hobbies and passions that bring fulfillment.

- Consider volunteering or mentoring to stay socially and mentally engaged.

- Develop new skills or start creative projects that provide joy and a sense of purpose.

In summary, menopause is a natural phase that should be embraced with knowledge, self-care, and a proactive mindset. By combining medical support, lifestyle modifications, and emotional well-being strategies, women can navigate menopause smoothly and rediscover their Ikigai—their reason for being.

(C) How Ikigai Can Help Women Embrace Menopause as an Opportunity for Reinvention and a New Beginning

Menopause is often perceived as a phase of decline, but in reality, it can be a powerful period of transformation, self-discovery, and renewal. The Japanese concept of *Ikigai*—which translates to "reason for being"—offers a guiding framework to help women navigate this transition with purpose and positivity. By aligning their passions, skills, societal contributions, and well-being, women can redefine this stage of life as a time of reinvention rather than limitation.

1. Reframing Menopause as a Gateway to Self-Discovery

Menopause is not just a biological event; it is a psychological and emotional shift that can open doors to new possibilities. Instead of viewing this transition as an end, women can use *Ikigai* to explore what truly brings them joy, meaning, and fulfillment.

- **Shifting the Mindset: From Loss to Opportunity**
  - **Freedom from Reproductive Responsibilities** – With menstruation and fertility behind them, women can embrace newfound autonomy and focus on personal growth.

  - **A Time for Self-Care** – Prioritizing health, well-being, and self-reflection becomes essential.

  - **Reassessing Priorities** – This is a time to evaluate what truly matters and remove societal pressures of youth and perfection.

  - **Celebrating Wisdom and Experience** – Years of life experience bring clarity, confidence, and a deeper understanding of oneself.

Ikigai in Menopause: Asking the Right Questions

- What activities make me lose track of time and bring me joy?

- How can I use my experience and wisdom to contribute to society?

- What strengths have I developed over the years, and how can I utilize them now?

- What lifestyle changes can I make to support my well-being and longevity?

2. Rediscovering Passions and Interests

Many women have spent decades prioritizing family, career, and societal expectations. Menopause offers a chance to reconnect with passions that may have been set aside.

How to Reignite Passions Through Ikigai

- **Exploring Creative Pursuits** – Painting, writing, music, or dance can serve as expressive outlets.

- **Travel and Exploration** – Exploring new places or engaging in cultural experiences can provide a sense of adventure.

- **Learning New Skills** – Taking up new hobbies or enrolling in courses can provide intellectual stimulation.

- **Entrepreneurship or Social Contribution** – Many women use this time to start businesses, mentor younger generations, or contribute to social causes.

Ikigai Exercise: Creating a Passion List

- Write down 10 things you loved doing as a child.

- List the things you've always wanted to try but never had the time for.

- Identify activities that bring you peace, joy, and excitement.

- Take small steps to incorporate these into your daily life.

3. Finding New Purpose Through Contribution and Meaningful Work

Many women struggle with a sense of loss during menopause, especially as children grow up or careers slow down. *Ikigai* emphasizes that life's purpose is deeply connected to how we contribute to the world around us.

Ways to Find New Purpose in This Stage

- **Mentorship & Coaching** – Sharing knowledge with younger women or mentoring in professional spaces.

- **Volunteering & Social Work** – Contributing to community projects or helping causes close to the heart.

- **Starting a Business or Side Hustle** – Utilizing years of experience to start an impactful venture.

- **Advocacy for Women's Health** – Spreading awareness about menopause, health, and self-care.

Ikigai Reflection: What Impact Can I Create?

- How can my life experiences help others?

- What problem in society do I feel passionate about solving?

- What kind of legacy do I want to leave behind?

4. Prioritizing Well-Being: The Foundation of a Fulfilling Life

Menopause often demands a shift in lifestyle to support long-term health. *Ikigai* teaches that true fulfillment comes from maintaining balance—physical, mental, and emotional well-being.

Integrating Well-Being into Daily Life

- **Mind-Body Connection** – Practicing yoga, tai chi, or mindfulness to maintain harmony.

- **Holistic Nutrition** – Eating for longevity with whole foods, anti-inflammatory diets, and hydration.

- **Movement and Strength** – Regular exercise to maintain muscle mass, bone density, and heart health.

- **Emotional Wellness** – Seeking therapy, journaling, and maintaining social connections.

- **Engaging in Joyful Activities** – Whether it's dancing, gardening, or reading, doing what feels good is key.

Ikigai Challenge: Create a Well-Being Plan

- What physical activities make me feel energized?

- What foods nourish me and support my long-term health?

- What relaxation practices can I implement daily?

- How can I create a daily routine that aligns with my well-being goals?

5. Strengthening Relationships and Community Bonds

Menopause can sometimes bring feelings of isolation, especially if a woman feels misunderstood. Strengthening relationships and building new connections can foster a sense of belonging and purpose.

Ways to Build Meaningful Relationships During This Phase

- **Deepening Family Bonds** – Spending quality time with loved ones and creating new traditions.

- **Connecting with Like-Minded Women** – Joining menopause support groups or women's circles.

- **Building New Friendships** – Exploring new social groups, clubs, or online communities.

- **Sharing Stories and Experiences** – Writing, blogging, or speaking to help normalize menopause conversations.

Ikigai Reflection: Who Are My People?

- Who uplifts and inspires me in my current phase of life?

- What kind of community do I want to build around me?

- How can I contribute positively to the relationships in my life?

6. Embracing Menopause as a Time for Personal Growth and Reinvention

This stage of life can be an opportunity to redefine who you are, let go of limiting beliefs, and embrace the best version of yourself. *Ikigai* offers a perspective that encourages growth, curiosity, and transformation.

Steps to Reinvention

- **Let Go of the Past** – Release outdated societal expectations and embrace personal evolution.

- **Visualize the Future** – Create a vision board or journal about the life you want post-menopause.

- **Stay Curious** – Keep learning, evolving, and challenging yourself.

- **Celebrate Aging** – View aging as a privilege and a journey of wisdom, not a decline.

- **Live with Intention** – Each day is an opportunity to align with your *Ikigai* and make life meaningful.

- **Ikigai Action Plan: Designing Your Next Chapter**
  - What do I want to experience in the next 10 years?

  - How can I continue growing mentally, emotionally, and spiritually?

  - What steps can I take today to align with my *Ikigai*?

In summary, menopause is not the end of youth—it is the beginning of wisdom, self-awareness, and purpose. By integrating Ikigai principles into daily life, women can turn this phase into a time of passion, fulfillment, and reinvention.

Instead of fearing change, embrace it. Instead of resisting aging, celebrate it. Instead of mourning what was, create what can be.

Menopause is not a loss. It's a transition into a powerful, fulfilling new phase of life—one guided by your Ikigai.

(D) Guided Ikigai Worksheet for Menopausal Women

Rediscovering Purpose, Wellness, and Joy in the Menopause Phase

Menopause is not just a biological transition—it is also a time for self-discovery, reinvention, and embracing new opportunities. This worksheet will help you reconnect with your purpose and create a fulfilling life aligned with Ikigai.

1. What You Love (Passion)

These are the activities, experiences, and pursuits that bring you joy and fulfillment.

- What makes you feel truly happy and alive at this stage in life?
  Example: Traveling, reading, spending time with grandchildren, volunteering, yoga, etc.

- What are the things you have always wanted to do but never had time for?
  Example: Learning a musical instrument, painting, writing a book, starting a business, etc.

- What moments make you feel most at peace and connected to yourself?
  Example: Early morning walks, meditation, cooking, listening to music, etc.

2. What You Are Good At (Vocation)

Your strengths, skills, and wisdom developed over the years.

- What are your biggest strengths that you have developed over time?

Example: Problem-solving, resilience, communication, leadership, creativity, etc.

- What are you naturally good at that could help others?
  Example: Mentoring, coaching, public speaking, writing, caregiving, etc.

- What do people often come to you for advice about?
  Example: Life guidance, career advice, parenting tips, emotional support, etc.

3. What the World (Your Community) Needs (Mission)

Ways you can contribute to others and find purpose.

- How can you inspire and support others during this phase of life?
  Example: Sharing your menopause journey, mentoring younger women, writing, public speaking, etc.

- What societal or community issues are close to your heart?
  Example: Women's health awareness, mental well-being, financial independence, education, etc.

- How can you leave a lasting impact or legacy?
  Example: Starting a social project, launching an online community, creating a blog, writing a book, etc.

4. What You Can Be Paid For (Profession)

Exploring financial independence and purpose-driven work.

- How can you use your skills and experience to create financial stability?
  Example: Coaching, consulting, teaching online, writing, entrepreneurship, freelancing, etc.

- Are there opportunities that align with your passions and skills?
  Example: Becoming a wellness coach, creating online courses, launching a creative business, etc.

- What kind of work would make you feel valued and energized at this stage?
  Example: Flexible work, remote opportunities, passion-based projects, etc.

Bringing It All Together: Your Ikigai Statement
Write a short paragraph combining the four elements (passion, vocation, mission, profession) to define your purpose.

Example:
"I love inspiring and mentoring women going through menopause. My years of experience in health and wellness allow me to share valuable insights with others. The world needs more awareness and support for menopausal women, and I can contribute through writing, coaching, and community-building. I can also turn my passion into a profession by offering workshops and online courses, allowing me to create a meaningful and financially sustainable career while empowering others."

Reflection Questions

- How do you see menopause as a new beginning rather than an end?
- What is one small step you can take today toward your Ikigai?
- What self-care habits can you integrate into your daily routine for better health and well-being?
- How can you embrace change with a positive mindset?

CHAPTER VI: MAKING THE RULE OF 80% (Hara Hachi Bu) APPLICABLE FOR WOMEN AT ALL STAGES OF LIFE.

"Eat breakfast like a king, lunch like a prince and

dinner like pauper"

-American Nutritionist Adelle Davis

(A) 80 % Rule in Ikigai

The 80% rule in Ikigai is a practice derived from the Okinawan lifestyle, which emphasizes moderation in eating. It is based on the phrase **"Hara Hachi Bu"**, which means **"eat until you are 80% full."**

How it Relates to Ikigai and Well-being:

1. **Longevity:** This habit prevents overeating and reduces the risk of obesity and related diseases. Okinawans known for their long lifespan, follow this rule as part of their daily routine.

2. **Mindful Eating:** It encourages awareness of hunger and satiety, aligning with the *Ikigai* philosophy of being present and enjoying life's simple pleasures.

3. **Energy Balance:** Overeating can lead to sluggishness, while stopping at 80% fullness keeps the body light and energetic.

4. **Sustainability:** This practice promotes food conservation, mindful consumption, and a sustainable lifestyle.

(B) How 80% Rule can be Beneficial for Adolescent Girls?

The 80% rule can be highly beneficial for adolescent girls especially as they go through puberty, hormonal changes, and increased nutritional demands.

1. **Prevents Overeating and Obesity Risks**
   - Adolescents often eat mindlessly due to stress, screen time, or pear influence.

   - The 80% role helps them develop a healthy relationship with food, reducing obesity risks.

2. **Balances Hormones and Reduces PCOS Risk**
   - Overeating, especially sugary and processed foods, can cause insulin resistance, a key factor in PCOS.

   - Practicing portion control helps maintain hormonal balance and menstrual regularity.

3. **Encourages Nutrient-Dense Eating for Growth**
   - Adolescence is a phase of rapid growth, requiring protein, calcium and healthy fats.

   - The 80% rule promotes mindful selection of nutrient-rich foods over junk food.

4. **Prevents Emotional and Binge Eating**
   - Many teenage girls struggle with body image issues and emotional eating.

   - Stopping at 80% fullness encourages intuitive eating habits and self-awareness.

5. **Improves Digestive Health:**
   - Overeating can cause bloating, sluggishness, and indigestion, which many teens experience.

   - Eating smaller, mindful portions support health and energy levels.

6. **Develops Lifelong Healthy Habits**
   - Teaching the 80% rule early helps girls carry this habit into adulthood, reducing risk of chronic diseases later in life.

(C) How 80% Rule of Ikigai Helps in Fertility, Hormonal Balance and Healthy Pregnancy?

Mindful eating, including practices like the 80% rule (Hara Hachi Bu), plays a significant role in infertility, hormonal balance, and a healthy pregnancy. Here is how:

1. **Supports Fertility**
   - **Regulates weight and BMI**: Being overweight or underweight can disrupt ovulation. Mindful eating helps maintain a healthy BMI, improving chances of conception.

   - **Reduces Insulin Resistance:** High insulin levels can interfere with ovulation, especially in conditions like PCOS. Eating in moderation helps regulate blood sugar.

   - **Boosts Nutrient Absorption:** Eating slowly and stopping at 80% fullness allows for better digestion and absorption for fertility-boosting nutrients like folate, iron and omega-3 fatty acids.

2. **Balances Hormones**
   - **Prevents Blood Sugar Spikes:** Overeating especially processed foods, causes glucose fluctuations, leading to hormonal imbalances (insulin, cortisol and estrogen).

   - **Supports Gut Health:** A well-balanced gut microbiome is essential for hormone metabolism. Mindful eating encourages a nutrient-dense, fiber-rich diet that nourishes gut bacteria.

- **Reduces Stress Hormones:** Chronic stress increases cortisol, which can negatively impact estrogen and progesterone levels. Eating mindfully lowers stress, promoting hormonal harmony.

3. **Ensures Healthy Pregnancy**
   - **Prevents Gestational Diabetes:** Eating until 80% full helps regulate weight gain and blood sugar, reducing the risk of gestational diabetes and hypertension.

   - **Enhances Digestive Health:** Pregnancy can slow digestion, leading to bloating and acid reflux. Eating slowly prevents overeating and reduces discomfort.

   - **Optimizes Fetal Nutrition:** Mindful eating prioritizes nutrient-dense foods that support fetal growth such as lean proteins, healthy fats, and leafy greens.

   - **Encourages a Balanced Relationship with Food:** Practicing mindful eating during pregnancy can help avoid emotional eating and carvings that may lead to excessive weight gain.

(D) How 80% Rule is Beneficial during Menopause

The 80% rule *(Hara Hachi Bu)* is especially beneficial during menopause, a phase marked by hormonal shifts, metabolic slowdown, and increased risk of chronic diseases. Here is how practicing mindful eating and stopping at 80% fullness can support in menopause.

1. **Helps Prevent Weight Gain and Obesity**
    - Metabolism naturally slows down after menopause, leading to weight gain if calorie isn't adjusted.

    - Overeating increases fat accumulation, especially around the abdomen, raising risks for diabetes and heart disease.

    - The 80% rule helps regulate calorie intake without strict dieting, promoting gradual weight maintenance.

2. **Regulates Blood Sugar and Prevents Diabetes**
    - Postmenopausal women are at a higher risk of insulin resistance due to lower estrogen levels.

    - Overeating, especially refined carbs, leads to blood sugar spikes and fat storage.

    - Stopping at 80% fullness prevents overeating, stabilizes blood sugar, and reduces diabetic risk.

3. **Reduces Risk of Hypertension and Heart Disease**
    - Estrogen helps protect heart health, but its decline post-menopause raises blood pressure and cholesterol levels.

- Overeating can lead to artery-clogging fats, increasing hypertension and heart disease risks.

- The 80% rule encourages portion control, reducing excess intake of sodium, unhealthy fats, and sugars.

4. Supports Digestion and Prevents Bloating

- Menopausal woman often experiences slower digestion, bloating and acidity reflux due to hormonal changes.

- Overeating worsens these issues, leading to discomfort and digestive distress.

- Eating smaller, mindful portions improves digestion and nutrient absorption.

5. Helps Balance Hormones and Reduce Hot Flashes

- Overeating can increase inflammation, which worsens hot flashes and mood swings.

- The 80% rule encourages mindful eating, reduces stress on the body and promoting hormone balance.

- It also helps prevent high estrogen dominance, which can lead to weight gain and mood fluctuations.

6. Supports Bone Health and Reduces Osteoporosis

- Calcium and Vitamin D absorption become less efficient after menopause.

- Eating beyond fullness often leads to a high-calorie, low nutrient diet, depriving bones of essential minerals.

- Mindful eating encourages nutrient-dense choices, supporting bone strength and joint health.

7. **Promoting Longevity and Healthy Aging**
   - Practicing the 80% rule is linked to longevity in Okinawan women, many of whom age gracefully with fewer chronic diseases.

   - Avoiding excess calorie intake reduces oxidative stress, preventing premature aging and inflammation-related diseases.

   - A balanced, moderate approach to eating supports vitality, mobility, and cognitive functions in later years.

In summary, making the 80% rule (Hara Hachi Bu) a universal guide for women at all stages of life – adolescence, reproductive years and menopause ties beautifully into the Ikigai philosophy of mindful living, helping women maintain hormonal balance, prevent diseases, and cultivate lifelong wellness.

CHAPTER VII: THE ROLE OF COMMUNITY AND SUPPORT SYSTEM

"Your health is your foundation,

and Ikigai is your compass—align them,

and you'll find the energy to live

a fulfilling and vibrant life."

-Anonymous

(A) The Role of Community and Support in Women's Health

1. Emotional Well-being and Stress Reduction

- Supportive relationships provide emotional stability, reducing stress and promoting mental health.

- Social bonds release oxytocin, which helps lower cortisol levels, mitigating anxiety and depression.

2. Accountability and Motivation

- A strong support system keeps women accountable for their health goals, making them more likely to follow through with commitments like exercise, healthy eating, and medical check-ups.

- Friends, families and support groups can offer encouragement and celebrate progress, reinforcing positive habits.

3.   Knowledge Sharing and Collective Wisdom

- Communities provide access to shared knowledge on health, nutrition and wellness, allowing women to make informed decisions.

- Mentors and experienced individuals can guide others on topics such as pregnancy, menopause, or disease prevention.

4.   Encouraging Healthy Habits Through Social Influence

- Being part of a health-conscious community, it fosters an environment where good habits like mindful eating and active living, become the norm.

- Social circles can influence dietary choices, exercise routines, and even medical adherence.

5.   Practical Assistance in Times of Need

- A support network helps during pregnancy, postpartum recovery, illness, or aging by providing hands-on care, guidance, and reassurance.

- Community resources, such as women's health groups, can bridge the gap in medical and emotional support.

6. Resilience and Coping Mechanisms

- Strong relationships provide emotional resilience, helping women navigate major life changes, including motherhood, menopause, or chronic illness.

- Women who engage in supportive networks report better coping strategies and a stronger sense of purpose.

7. Spiritual and Psychological Nourishment

- A sense of belonging and connection contributes to overall life satisfaction and inner peace, aligning with the Ikigai philosophy.

- Religious and mindfulness-based communities can offer spiritual support, enhancing mental well-being.

8. Economic and Professional Support

- Financial and career-related support, such as networking opportunities or shared childcare responsibilities, empowers women to pursue personal and professional growth.

- Women's collectives and cooperative groups provide avenues for skill-building and economic independence.

9. Intergenerational Learning and Support

- Relationships with different generations foster wisdom exchange, benefitting younger women with championship and purpose.

- Elders provide traditional knowledge, while younger generations introduce modern health approaches.

10. Enhancing Longevity and Overall Well-being

- Studies show that women with strong social connections live longer and experience better physical and mental health.

- The Ikigai principle emphasizes interconnectedness, reinforcing the role of social bonds in achieving a fulfilling and healthy life.

(B) How Finding One's Ikigai Enriches the Community

1. **Fostering a Sense of Purpose in Others**

   - When a woman discovers her *Ikigai*, she naturally inspires those around her to pursue their own passions and purpose.

   - This creates a ripple effect where more individuals engage in meaningful activities, enriching the community.

2. **Strengthening Social Bonds**

   - Living with *Ikigai* encourages dipper and more fulfilling relationships, fostering a culture of connection and support.

   - It enhances empathy and kindness, making communities more inclusive and harmonious.

3. **Encouraging Health and Well-being**

   - Women aligned with their *Ikigai* are more likely to maintain good health habits, setting an example for others.

   - They can become mentors, advocates, or wellness leaders, promoting healthy lifestyles in their communities.

4. Sharing Skills and Knowledge

- A woman who embraces her Ikigai often shares her expertise, whether in health, education, business, or the arts.

- This leads to skill-building initiatives, mentorship programs, and educational opportunities for others.

5. Building Resilience Support Networks

- *Ikigai* offers a deep sense of belonging, leading to stronger community networks where members uplift and empower one another.

- Women with a clear purpose contribute to initiatives like support groups, advocacy movements, and volunteer work.

6. Enhancing Economic and Social Development

- By turning their passion into meaningful work, women contribute to the local economy, whether through entrepreneurship, social enterprises, or creative industries.

- Purpose-driven women often initiate projects that address community needs, such as healthcare access, environmental sustainability, or education.

7. **Providing Intergenerational Wisdom**

- When women live with *Ikegai*, they become vessels of wisdom, passing down knowledge and cultural values to younger generations.

- This strengthens the community's collective identity and resilience over time.

8. **Creating a Culture of Joy and Fulfillment**

- People who find meaning in their daily lives radiate positivity, making the community a more uplifting place.

- They contribute to social and cultural activities that bring people together, from wellness circles to artistic endeavors.

9. **Encouraging Collective Growth**

- A community thrives when individuals are engaged in meaningful work that aligns with their passions and values.

- Women living with *Ikigai* contribute by encouraging teamwork, collaboration and shared success.

10. **Leaving a Lasting Legacy**

- A woman who fully embraces her *Ikigai* doesn't just improve her own life – she leaves a positive impact that continues for generations.

- Whether through mentorship, innovation, or leadership, her contributions shape the future of her community.

In summary, by aligning personal purpose with communal well-being, woman can transform their communities into thriving, supportive, and empowered spaces.

CHAPTER VIII: PERSONALISED IKIGAI IN WOMEN'S HEALTH

Discover your purpose, overcome challenges,

and make better choices

about your personalized health through Ikigai

-Anonymous

In the chapter **"Personalized Ikigai in Women's Health,"** identifying and living with *Ikigai* can be broken down into structured steps that align with different stages of a woman's life—adolescence, reproductive age, and menopause. This ensures that Ikigai remains a guiding force throughout various phases of health and well-being.

1. Understanding Ikigai in Women's Health

Ikigai (生き甲斐) is a Japanese concept meaning *"reason for being."* It is the intersection of:

- **What you love** (passion)
- **What you are good at** (vocation)
- **What the world needs** (mission)
- **What you can be paid for** (profession)

In the context of women's health, **Ikigai** is about **aligning lifestyle choices, self-care, and purpose** to maintain physical, mental, and emotional well-being.

2. How to Identify Your Ikigai

Women at different life stages can **find their personalized Ikigai** by reflecting on key questions:

Adolescence (Building Foundations)

- What excites you the most about life?
- What activities make you feel alive?
- What skills do you enjoy developing?
- How can you take care of your body and mind while pursuing your interests?

Reproductive Age (Balancing Health, Career, and Family)

- How do you balance personal well-being with career and relationships?
- What lifestyle choices energize you?
- What habits keep you physically and mentally strong?
- How can you create time for personal growth amidst responsibilities?

Menopause (Rediscovering Self & New Purpose)

- What legacy do you want to leave behind?
- How can you focus on health and joy in this phase?
- What hobbies or passions do you want to reignite?
- What are new ways to contribute to society while maintaining a healthy lifestyle?

3. Living with Ikigai: Practical Strategies

Once identified, **living with Ikigai** requires a holistic approach:

Physical Health (Movement & Nutrition)

- Find an enjoyable exercise routine (Yoga, Walking, Strength Training).
- Eat nourishing foods that support hormonal balance (Green tea, Omega-3 fatty acids, Whole foods).
- Maintain gut health (fermented foods, hydration, mindful eating).

Mental Well-being (Mindfulness & Stress Management)

- Practice daily gratitude and meditation.
- Engage in creative hobbies (painting, music, writing).
- Foster positive relationships that uplift mental and emotional health.

Preventive Health Care

- Regular check-ups and screenings.
- Understanding body changes (menstrual cycles, pregnancy, menopause symptoms).
- Seeking holistic and medical guidance for well-being.

Purpose & Growth

- Setting personal and professional goals.
- Engaging in lifelong learning.
- Teaching, mentoring, or giving back to the community.

4. Creating a Personalized Ikigai Plan

Women can create a **Personalized Ikigai Map** to help them stay aligned:

Aspect	Your Personal Answer
What do you love?	(Fill in your passion)
What are you good at?	(Your strengths & skills)
What does the world need from you?	(Your role in family/society)
What can you be paid for?	(Career & financial stability)

Aspect	Your Personal Answer
Health Priorities	(Physical & mental well-being goals)
Daily Ikigai Practice	(Rituals & habits to nurture purpose).

5. Final Thoughts: Ikigai as a Lifelong Companion

Ikigai is not a **one-time discovery** but a **continuous journey**. Women's health and priorities change over time, and so does their *Ikigai*. The key is to stay adaptable, listen to the body, and embrace **Ikigai-driven living** at every stage.

By incorporating **Ikigai in Women's Health**, women can lead a **balanced, joyful, and fulfilling life**—physically, mentally, and emotionally.

CHAPTER IX: CULTURAL WISDOM MEETS MODERN SCIENCE

Traditional wisdom is not a relic of the past,

it is the foundation upon which

modern science builds its greatest advancements.

-Anonymous

The interaction between traditional wisdom and modern medical practices in gynecology presents a unique opportunity to offer holistic, patient-centered care. Historically, women's health has been shaped by cultural beliefs, ancient healing methods, and natural remedies, many of which align with modern scientific findings. By merging cultural wisdom with evidence-based medicine, we can create a purpose-driven approach to gynecological treatment that honors tradition while leveraging modern advancements.

1. Traditional Wisdom & Gynecology: A Timeless Foundation

Throughout history, different cultures have developed unique approaches to women's health, using herbal medicine, dietary practices, and mind-body techniques to manage reproductive health. Some of these traditional practices remain relevant today:

- ✓ **Ayurveda (India)** – Balances *doshas* for menstrual health, menopause, and pregnancy through food, yoga, and herbs like **Shatavari** (supports fertility) and **Ashwagandha** (reduces stress).

- ✓ **Traditional Chinese Medicine (TCM)** – **Uses acupuncture, herbal formulas, and Qi (energy)**

flow to regulate cycles, alleviate PCOS, and support postpartum recovery.

✓ **Japanese Kampo Medicine** – Includes remedies like **Tochuu (Eucommia Bark)** and **Kampo herbal formulas** to support hormonal balance and uterine health.

✓ **Indigenous & Folk Medicine** – Many communities use **rituals, massage therapies, and dietary principles** to enhance **fertility, postpartum healing, and menopause comfort**.

Many of these approaches align with modern science, emphasizing gut health, hormone balance, stress management, and holistic well-being.

2. Modern Medical Science: Evidence-Based Advancements in Gynecology

While traditional methods provide **long-standing insights**, modern gynecology **advances treatment through scientific validation**. Key developments include:

✓ **Hormonal Therapies** – MHT (Menopause Hormone Therapy) for managing **perimenopause/menopause, and hormonal imbalances**.

✓ **Minimally Invasive Surgeries** – Laparoscopy and robotic-assisted procedures for **fibroids, endometriosis, and hysterectomies**.

✓ **Genetic & Hormone Testing** – Personalized treatment plans using **DNA-based diagnostics, AMH (Anti-Müllerian Hormone) tests for fertility**, and PCOS screening.

✓ **Microbiome & Gut Health Research** – Understanding **vaginal microbiota and gut-brain-**

hormone connections to prevent infections and regulate cycles.

- ✓ **Mind-Body Science** – Studies confirm that **meditation, acupuncture, and yoga** improve outcomes in pregnancy, fertility, and menopause, aligning with traditional practices.

Rather than rejecting traditional wisdom, modern medicine is increasingly validating its benefits.

3. A Purpose-Driven Approach to Gynecological Treatment

A **purpose-driven approach** integrates the best of **both worlds**—leveraging **scientific advancements** while **embracing the wisdom of tradition**. This means:

Holistic, Patient-Centered Care

- ✓ Addressing **not just symptoms but lifestyle, emotions, and cultural beliefs**.

- ✓ Encouraging **dietary modifications, stress management, and holistic support** alongside medical treatments.

- ✓ Using **scientifically backed natural supplements** (e.g., omega-3 fatty acids, probiotics), **prevention over cure** instead of **treating diseases reactively**, a purpose-driven approach **prioritizes prevention**.

- ✓ Encouraging **early detection screenings, period tracking for hormonal imbalances**, and **gut health optimization**.

- ✓ Empowering women with **nutritional knowledge, lifestyle interventions, and alternative therapies** to avoid invasive treatments.

Mental & Emotional Well-Being in Women's Health

✓ Gynecological disorders often have **a psychosomatic component**. Stress, trauma, and lifestyle play a role in **PCOS, menstrual irregularities, and infertility**.

✓ A purpose-driven approach **considers mental well-being, counseling, meditation, and community support** as part of treatment.

✓ For example, research shows **mindfulness and acupuncture** can improve fertility success rates and reduce menopause symptoms.

4. Case Study: Combining Tradition & Modern Science in Practice

Consider a woman with **PCOS (Polycystic Ovary Syndrome)**. A **purpose-driven approach** would involve:

- **Traditional Insights:**
  - Ayurveda suggests balancing *Kapha dosha* with diet (warm foods, less dairy/sugar).
  - Chinese Medicine recommends **acupuncture** and **herbal teas** to regulate cycles.
  - Yoga & breathing exercises improve **insulin sensitivity and stress response.**

- **Modern Medical Approach:**
  - Metformin or Inositol for insulin resistance.
  - Hormonal therapy if needed.
  - Regular **ultrasound & blood tests** to monitor ovarian health.

- **Integrated Plan:**
  By **combining these approaches**, the woman experiences **improved cycle regularity, weight management, and mental clarity**, while avoiding excessive medications.

5. Bridging the Gap: How Doctors Can Integrate Both Approaches

For a **true fusion of cultural wisdom and modern science**, healthcare professionals should:

- **Respect cultural preferences** – Acknowledge a patient's belief system while guiding them toward science-backed interventions.

- **Prescribe complementary therapies** – Suggest **meditation, acupuncture, or diet changes** along with medications when appropriate.

- **Stay updated on integrative medicine** – Recognizing that **ancient wisdom has merit when combined with scientific evidence**.

- **Educate & empower patients** – Teaching women how **nutrition, stress management, and lifestyle habits** impact reproductive health.

CHAPTER X: CONCLUSION AND CALL TO ACTION: EMBRACING YOUR HEALTH AND IKEGAI

"Ikigai isn't just about longevity;

it's about thriving at every age,

honouring your body, mind,

and soul in the process."

-Anonymous

According to Japanese philosophy, everyone has an ***Ikigai.*** Some people have found their ***Ikigai***, while others are still in a process of identifying, though they carry it within them in hidden form.

1. **Reflect on Your Personal Ikigai**

    - Take time to discover what truly brings your joy, fulfillment and purpose.

    - Journal about activities that make you feel alive and connected to your inner self.

2. **Prioritize Holistic Health**

    - View health as a lifelong journey that integrates physical, mental and emotional well-being.

    - Adopt small, sustainable lifestyle changes that align with your personal Ikigai.

3. Nourish Your Body with Intension

- Apply the ***Hara Hashi Bu*** (80%rule) for mindful eating and hormonal balance.

- Choose nutrient-dense, whole food that support your reproductive health and overall well-being.

4. Build Resilience Through Ikigai

- Face life's challenges with the mindset that your purpose gives you strength.

- Use Ikigai as an anker during difficult phases like motherhood, menopause or career transitions.

5. Strengthen Your Community and Support System

- Surround yourself with people who uplift, inspire, and support your health goals.

- Engage in social circles, women groups, or mentorship programs that align with your values.

6. Move with Joy and Intension

- Incorporate movement that you enjoy, whether it is yoga, dance, walking, or strength training.

- Focus on consistency rather than perfection.

7. **Practice Rest and Stress Management**

- Prioritize quality sleep and relaxation techniques like meditation and deep breathing.

- Reduce stress by setting boundaries and engaging in self-care without guilt.

8. **Take Action – Start Small, Stay Committed**

- Identify one small change you can make today that aligns with your health and Ikigai.

- Track your progress and celebrate your wins, no matter how small.

9. **Inspire and Lift Other Women**

- Share your journey and encourage other women to prioritize their health and purpose.

- Advocate for women's well-being in your community, work place, or social circles.

10. **Your Health, Your Ikigai – Begin Today!**

- There is no perfect time to start – begin now, wherever you are.

- Every step toward better health brings you closer to a life of meaning, joy, and vitality.

- Whatever you do, don't ever retire from doing meaningful activities.

APPENDIX

IKIGAI AND WOMEN'S HEALTH WORKBOOK

A Practical Guide to Living with Purpose and Well-being

Section 1: Discovering Your Ikigai

Exercise 1: Self-Reflection on Purpose

- What activities bring you joy?

- What are you naturally good at?

- How do you contribute to others?

- What does the world need that aligns with your strength

(Write down your thoughts in each category and find the overlap – this is your *Ikigai*.)

Exercise 2: Journaling Prompts

- When I feel most alive?

- What values guide my decisions?

- What kind of legacy do I want to leave behind?

Section 2: Prioritizing Holistic Health

Exercise 3: Health Goals & Tracker

- List three specific health goals (e.g., improving sleep, eating mindfully, managing stress).

- Break them into small, actionable steps (e.g., sleep by 10 pm, eat until 80% full, practice deep breathing).

- Use a weekly tracker to monitor progress.

Section 3: Mindful Eating and *Hara Hachi Bu*

Exercise 4: Food Awareness Journal

- Track what you eat, your portion size, and how you feel afterward. (e.g., **Lunch** – Salad + Rice – Fullness level: 7 = Energized feel. **Dinner** – Pasta + Bread – Fullness level: 9 = Bloated feel.)

- Identify patterns – do you eat out of hunger, stress, or habit?

- List ways to implement *Hara Hachi Bu* in daily life.

Section 4: Strengthening Your Support System

Exercise 5: Community & Connection Map

- Who support your health journey? (List mentors, friends, family, groups).

- How can you strengthen these connections?

- Identify one person to check in with weekly for motivation.
  - Schedule a health check-in with a friend.

- o Join an online or local women's wellness group.

Section 5: Daily Practices for a Balanced Life

Exercise 6: Daily Ikigai Checklist

- o Did I engage in something meaningful today?

- o Did I nourish my body mindfully?

- o Did I rest and recharge?

- o Did I nurture my relationships?

Final Call to Action: Your Commitment

Write a short letter to yourself, committing to your health and *Ikigai* journey.

"Dear (your name), I am committed to prioritizing my well-being because……………"

- o Sign and date your commitment.

CHAPTER XI: REFERENCES

1. *García, Héctor; Miralles, Francesc (2017). Ikigai: The Japanese Secret to a Long and Happy Life. Penguin Books. ISBN 978-0143130727.*

2. *^ Jump up to:[a][b] "Ikigai: The Japanese Secret to a Joyful Life". The Government of Japan - JapanGov -. 2024-02-29. Retrieved 2024-04-13.*

3. *^ Schippers, Michaéla (2017-06-16). IKIGAI: Reflection on Life Goals Optimizes Performance and Happiness. Erasmus Research Institute of Management, Erasmus University Rotterdam. ISBN 978-90-5892-484-1. Archived from the original on 2021-02-04. Retrieved 2020-03-05.*

4. *^ Mathews, Gordon (1996). "The Stuff of Dreams, Fading: Ikigai and "The Japanese Self"". Ethos. 24 (4): 718–747. doi:10.1525/eth.1996.24.4.02a00060. ISSN 0091-2131. JSTOR 640520.*

5. *^ Schippers, Michaéla C.; Ziegler, Niklas (2019-12-13). "Life Crafting as a Way to Find Purpose and Meaning in Life". Frontiers in Psychology. 10: 2778. doi:10.3389/fpsyg.2019.02778. ISSN 1664-1078. PMC 6923189. PMID 31920827.*

6. *^ Kumano, Michiko (2018-06-01). "On the Concept of Well-Being in Japan: Feeling Shiawase as Hedonic Well-Being and Feeling Ikigai as Eudaimonic Well-Being". Applied Research in Quality of Life. 13 (2): 419–433. doi:10.1007/s11482-017-9532-9. ISSN 1871-2576. S2CID 149162906.*

7. *^ Nakanishi, N (1999-05-01). "'Ikigai' in older Japanese people". Age and Ageing. 28 (3): 323–324. doi:10.1093/ageing/28.3.323. ISSN 1468-2834. PMID 10475874.*

8. *^ Okuzono, Sakurako S.; Shiba, Koichiro; Kim, Eric S.; Shirai, Kokoro; Kondo, Naoki; Fujiwara, Takeo; Kondo, Katunori; Lomas, Tim; Trudel-Fitzgerald, Claudia; Kawachi, Ichiro; VanderWeele, Tyler J. (2022). "Ikigai and subsequent health and wellbeing among Japanese*

*older adults: Longitudinal outcome-wide analysis". The Lancet Regional Health - Western Pacific. **21**: 100391. doi:10.1016/j.lanwpc.2022.100391. PMC 8814687. PMID 35141667.*

9. ^ *Miyazaki, Junji; Shirai, Kokoro; Kimura, Takashi; Ikehara, Satoyo; Tamakoshi, Akiko; Iso, Hiroyasu (2022). "Purpose in life (Ikigai) and employment status in relation to cardiovascular mortality: the Japan Collaborative Cohort Study". BMJ Open. **12** (10): e059725. doi:10.1136/bmjopen-2021-059725. PMC 9557793. PMID 36216422.*

10. ^ *Wilkes, Juliet; Garip, Gulcan; Kotera, Yasuhiro; Fido, Dean (2023). "Can Ikigai Predict Anxiety, Depression, and Well-being?". International Journal of Mental Health and Addiction. **21** (5): 2941–2953. doi:10.1007/s11469-022-00764-7. PMC 8887802. PMID 35250405.*

11. . Ten VT. Menstrual hygiene: A neglected condition for the achievement of several millennium development goals. *Europe External Policy Advisors.* 2007. [Last retrieved on 2014 Aug 09]. Available from: http://www.eepa.be/wcm/component/option,com_r emository/func, startdown/id, 26/

12. 4. Kumar A, Srivastava K. Cultural and social practices regarding menstruation among adolescent girls. *Soc Work Public Health.* 2011; 26:594–604. [PubMed] [Google Scholar]

13. 5. UNICEF. Bangladesh: Tackling menstrual hygiene taboos. Sanitation and Hygiene Case Study No. 10. 2008. [Last accessed on 2014 Aug 12]. Available from: http://www.unicef.org/wash/files/10_case_study_B ANGLADESH_4web.pdf .

14. 6. Sadiq MA, Salih AA. Knowledge and practice of adolescent females about menstruation in Baghdad. *J Gen Pract.* 2013; 2:138. [Google Scholar]

15. 7. Morley W. Common myths about your period. 2014. [Last accessed on 2014 Aug 12]. Available from: http://www.womenshealth.answers.com/menstruati on/common-myths-about-your-period .

16. Poureslami M, Osati-Ashtiani F. Assessing knowledge, attitudes, and behavior of adolescent girls in suburban districts of Tehran about dysmenorrhoea and menstrual hygiene. *J Int Womens Stud.* 2002; 3:51–61. [Google Scholar]

17. SOS Childrens' Village. Social taboos damage the health of girls and women. 2014. [Last accessed on 2014 Aug 12]. Available from: http://www.soschildrensvillages.org.uk/news/blog/socia l-taboos-damage-the-health-of-girls-and-women .

18. Clinical Practice on menopause – Indian Menopause Society.
19. Journal of Mid Life Health.
20. Menopause and MHT in 2024: addressing the key controversies – an International Menopause Society White Paper. (https://doi.org/10.1080/13697137.2024.2394950)
21. Dinnerstein L, Dudley EC, Hopper JL et. al. A prospective population-based study of menopause symptoms. Obstet. Gynecol 2000; 96:351.
22. Woods NF, Mitchell ES. Symptoms during the menopause: prevalence, severity and significance in women's lives. Am J Med 2005; 118 suppl 12 B: 14.
23.National Institute of Health State-of-the-Science Conference Statement: management of menopause-related symptoms. Ann Intern Med 2005; 142:1003.
24. Kronenberg F. Hot flashes: epidemiology and physiology. Ann N Y Acad Sci 1090; 592:52.
25.McKinley SM. The normal menopause transition: an overview. Maturitas 1996; 23:137.
26.Cohen LS, Soars CN, Joffe H. Diagnosis and management of mood disorders during menopause transition. Am J Med 2005; 118 suppl 12B:93.
27.Freedom RR, Roehrs TA. Sleep disturbances in menopause. Menopause 2007; 14:826.
28.The NAMS 2017 Hormone Therapy Position Statement Advisory Panel. The 2017 hormone therapy position statement

of the North American Menopause Society. Menopause 2017; 24:728.

29.Steingold KA, Laufer L, Chetkowski RJ, et.al. Treatment of hot flashes with transdermal estradiol administration. J Clin Endocrinol Metab 1985; 61:627.

30.Nelson HD. Commonly used types of postmenopausal oestrogen for treatment of hot flashes: scientific review. JAWA 2004; 291:1610.

31.North American Menopause Society. The 2012 hormone position statement of: The North American Menopause Society. Menopause 2012; 19:257.

32. Sood R, Faubion SS, Kuhle CL et.al prescribing Menopause Therapy: an evidence-based approach. Int. J Women's Health 2014; 6:47.

33.Udoff L, Langenberg P, Adashi EY. Combined Continuous Hormone Replacement Therapy: a critical review. Obstet Gynecol 1995; 86:306.

34.ACOG Practice Bulletin No. 141: management of menopausal symptoms. Obstet Gynecol. 2014;123(1):202-216.

35.Bakour SH, Williamson J. Latest evidence on using hormone therapy in the menopause. Obstet Gynecol, 2014.

36.The 2022 hormone therapy position statement of the North American Menopause Society. Menopause (New York). 2022;29(7):767-794.

Article Google Scholar

36. Jones, D. C., Vigfusdottir, T. H., & Lee, Y. (2004). Body image and the appearance culture among adolescent girls and boys: An examination of friend conversations, peer criticism, appearance magazines, and the internalization of appearance ideals. *Journal of Adolescent Research, 19*(3), 323–339. https://doi.org/10.1177/0743558403258847

Article Google Scholar

37.Jones, L. R., Fries, E., & Danish, S. J. (2007). Gender and ethnic differences in body image and opposite sex figure preferences of rural adolescents. *Body Image, 4*(1), 103–108. https://doi.org/10.1016/j.bodyim.2006.11.005

Article PubMed PubMed Central Google Scholar

38.. Kapidzic, S., & Herring, S. C. (2015). Race, gender, and self-presentation in teen profile photographs. *New Media & Society, 17*(6), 958–976. https://doi.org/10.1177/1461444813520301

Article Google Scholar

39.Keyes, K. M., Gary, D., O'Malley, P. M., Hamilton, A., & Schulenberg, J. (2019). Recent increases in depressive symptoms among U.S. adolescents: Trends from 1991 to 2018. *Social Psychiatry and Psychiatric Epidemiology, 54*(8), 987–996. https://doi.org/10.1007/s00127-019-01697-8

Article PubMed PubMed Central Google Scholar

40.Kim, H. M. (2020). What do others' reactions to body posting on Instagram tell us? The effects of social media comments on viewers' body image perception. *New Media & Society*. https://doi.org/10.1177/1461444820956368

ArticleGoogle Scholar

41.Pfeifer, J.H.; Allen, N.B. Puberty Initiates Cascading Relationships Between Neurodevelopmental, Social, and Internalizing Processes Across Adolescence. *Biol. Psychiatry* **2021**, *89*, 99–108. [**Google Scholar**] [**CrossRef**]
42.Guo, N.; Robakis, T.; Miller, C.; Butwick, A. Prevalence of Depression Among Women of Reproductive Age in the United States. *Obstet. Gynecol.* **2018**, *131*, 671–679. [**Google Scholar**] [**CrossRef**]
43.Angold, A.; Costello, E.J.; Erkanli, A.; Worthman, C.M. Pubertal Changes in Hormone Levels and Depression in Girls. *Psychol. Med.* **1999**, *29*, 1043–1053. [**Google Scholar**] [**CrossRef**] [**PubMed**]

44.Gordon, J.L.; Eisenlohr-Moul, T.A.; Rubinow, D.R.; Schrubbe, L.; Girdler, S.S. Naturally Occurring Changes in Estradiol Concentrations in the Menopause Transition Predict Morning Cortisol and Negative Mood in Perimenopausal Depression. *Clin. Psychol. Sci.* **2016**, *4*, 919–935. [**Google Scholar**] [**CrossRef**] [**PubMed**]

45.Bennett, H.A.; Einarson, A.; Taddio, A.; Koren, G.; Einarson, T.R. Prevalence of Depression during Pregnancy: Systematic Review. *Obstet. Gynecol.* **2004**, *103*, 698–709. [**Google Scholar**] [**CrossRef**] [**PubMed**]

46.Bloch, M.; Schmidt, P.J.; Danaceau, M.; Murphy, J.; Nieman, L.; Rubinow, D.R. Effects of Gonadal Steroids in Women with a History of Postpartum Depression. *Am. J. Psychiatry* **2000**, *157*, 924–930. [**Google Scholar**] [**CrossRef**]

47.Georgakis, M.K.; Thomopoulos, T.P.; Diamantaras, A.-A.; Kalogirou, E.I.; Skalkidou, A.; Daskalopoulou, S.S.; Petridou, E.T. Association of Age at Menopause and Duration of Reproductive Period with Depression After Menopause: A Systematic Review and Meta-Analysis. *JAMA Psychiatry* **2016**, *73*, 139–149. [**Google Scholar**] [**CrossRef**]

48.Freeman, E.W.; Sammel, M.D.; Liu, L.; Gracia, C.R.; Nelson, D.B.; Hollander, L. Hormones and Menopausal Status as Predictors of Depression in Women in Transition to Menopause. *Arch. Gen. Psychiatry* **2004**, *61*, 62–70. [**Google Scholar**] [**CrossRef**]

Gordon, J.L.; Peltier, A.; Grummisch, J.A.; Sykes Tottenham, L. Estradiol Fluctuation, Sensitivity to Stress, and Depressive Symptoms in the Menopause Transition: A Pilot Study. *Front. Psychol.* **2019**, *10*, 1319. [**Google Scholar**] [**CrossRef**]

49.Gordon, J.L.; Rubinow, D.R.; Eisenlohr-Moul, T.A.; Leserman, J.; Girdler, S.S. Estradiol Variability, Stressful Life Events, and the Emergence of Depressive Symptomatology during the Menopausal Transition. *Menopause* **2016**, *23*, 257–266. [**Google Scholar**] [**CrossRef**]

50.Almeida, O.P.; Lautenschlager, N.; Vasikaram, S.; Leedman, P.; Flicker, L. Association between Physiological Serum Concentration of Estrogen and the Mental Health of Community-Dwelling Postmenopausal Women Age 70 Years and over. *Am. J. Geriatr. Psychiatry* **2005**, *13*, 142–149. [**Google Scholar**] [**CrossRef**]

51.Ryan, J.; Burger, H.G.; Szoeke, C.; Lehert, P.; Ancelin, M.-L.; Henderson, V.W.; Dennerstein, L. A Prospective Study of the Association between Endogenous Hormones and Depressive Symptoms in Postmenopausal Women. *Menopause* **2009**, *16*, 509–517. [**Google Scholar**] [**CrossRef**]

52.Gudipally, P.R.; Sharma, G.K. *Premenstrual Syndrome*; StatPearls Publishing: Treasure Island, FL, USA, 2022. [**Google Scholar**]

53.Roomruangwong, C.; Carvalho, A.F.; Comhaire, F.; Maes, M. Lowered Plasma Steady-State Levels of Progesterone Combined with Declining Progesterone Levels During the Luteal Phase Predict Peri-Menstrual Syndrome and Its Major Subdomains. *Front. Psychol.* **2019**, *10*, 2446. [**Google Scholar**] [**CrossRef**] [**PubMed**]

54.Ford, O.; Lethaby, A.; Roberts, H.; Mol, B.W.J. Progesterone for Premenstrual Syndrome. *Cochrane Database Syst. Rev.* **2012**, *2012*, CD003415. [**Google Scholar**] [**CrossRef**] [**PubMed**]

55.Lovick, T.A.; Guapo, V.G.; Anselmo-Franci, J.A.; Loureiro, C.M.; Faleiros, M.C.M.; Del Ben, C.M.; Brandão, M.L. A Specific Profile of Luteal Phase Progesterone Is Associated with the Development of Premenstrual Symptoms. *Psychoneuroendocrinology* **2017**, *75*, 83–90. [**Google Scholar**] [**CrossRef**] [**PubMed**]

Previous Books Published in the Series, "Women's Health"

All books are available on Amazon.in as well as on Amazon.com.

Universal Link:

https://relinks.me/B0BW6ZVMXY

1. Preconception Care Makes a Difference

"Preconception Care and Counselling is the window of opportunity to tackle all unhealthy maternal problems resulting in favorable environment for the growth of embryo/fetus."

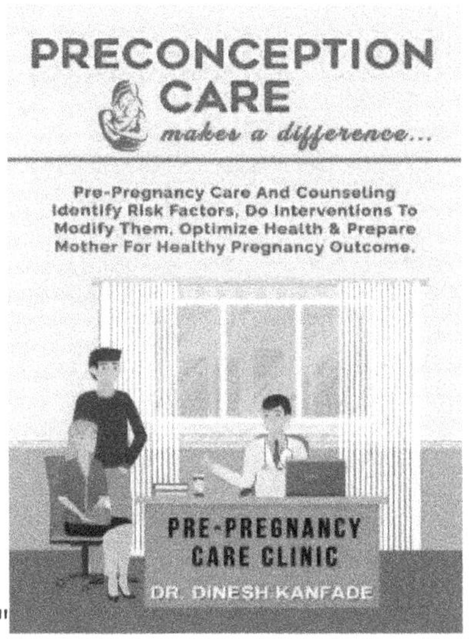

2. Understanding Menopause

"The biggest achievement of the last century is greater longevity that has resulted in an increased aged population worldwide. But the advantage of increased longevity is only when it is translated into healthy aging. Discover the secrets for understanding and managing menopause, thereby improving quality of life with this comprehensive updated guide."

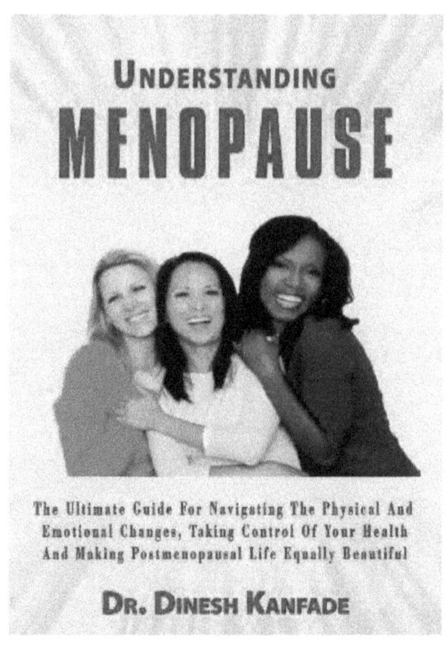

3. Heart and Bone Health

"We are living in aged population worldwide. It is obvious that women live significant part of their life after menopause. The ovaries of long years of dedicated service, have not the ability of retiring gracefully. But because of estrogen deficiency, ovaries become irritable and transmits this irritation to various organs of the body resulting in non-communicable diseases such as cardiovascular disease and osteoporosis. The advantage of increased longevity is only when it is translated into healthy aging. With a healthy lifestyle and understanding the pathophysiology of cardiovascular disease and osteoporosis in postmenopausal women, not only years will be added to increase the lifespan, but the extra years added will be of good quality. Discover the secretes of managing heart and bone health in postmenopausal women, thereby improving quality of life with this comprehensive guide."

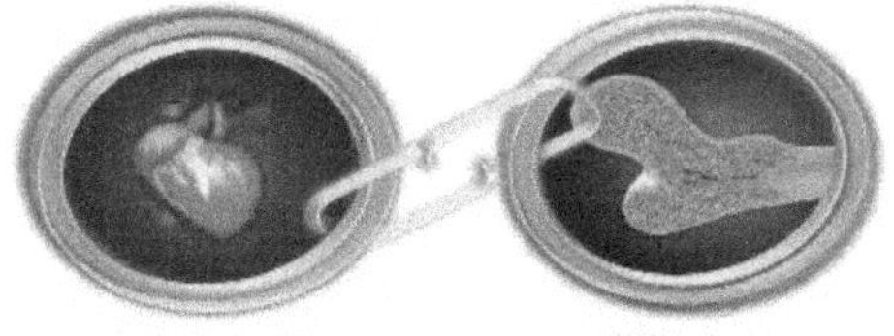

4. Embracing Postmenopausal Intimacy

"The postmenopausal phase, with its unique challenges and opportunities stands as a testament to the resilience of human intimacy. It is within this period of transformation that find an invitation to redefine and to rediscover physical closeness. Don't miss out on the transformative wisdom within these pages. Embrace the journey towards vibrant and fulfilling postmenopausal intimacy."

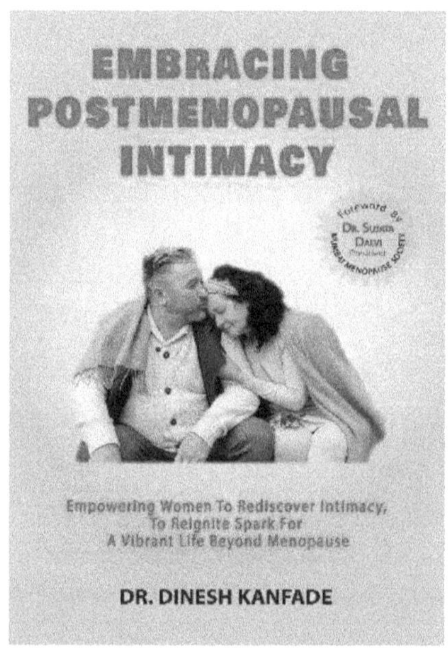

5. Menstrual Health and Hygiene

Unlock the secrets to optimal menstrual health and hygiene in this comprehensive guide.
From debunking myths to empowering insights, this book offers practical tips and evidence-based strategies for every stage of menstruation.

Whether you are seeking solutions for menstrual discomfort, navigating hygiene products or simply aiming for a healthier menstrual cycle, this book has covered everything you want in relation to menstruation.

Together, let us embark on this journey of enlightment, guided by the wisdom contained within these pages.

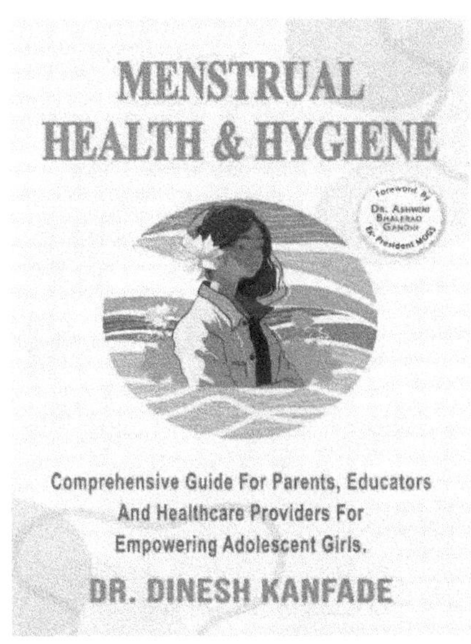

6. **The Silent Struggles: Understanding Women's Mental Health**

Mental health is often a quiet battle, and for women, it is a journey through the unique challenges at every stage of life.

The book is a comprehensive exploration of the emotional and psychological hurdles women face- from adolescence, through their reproductive years, to menopause.

The recurrence of heinous acts such as recent physical and sexual assault of junior doctor R. G. Kar Medical College Kolkata (August 2024), the infamous Nirbhaya case (2012) and many others suggest several concerning ground realities.

This book offers a profound understanding of how social, cultural and biological factors shape a woman's mental health.

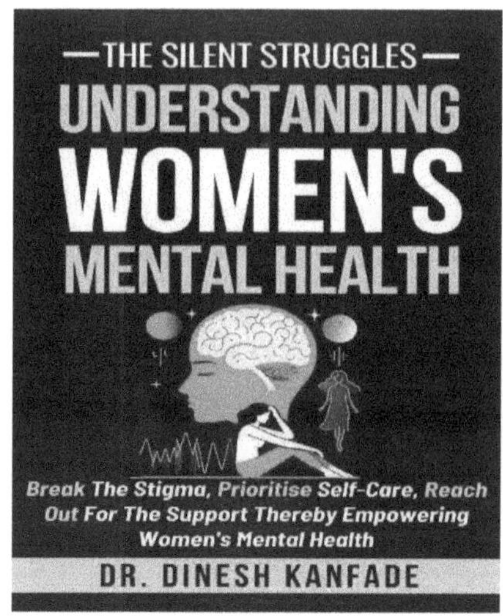

7. Nurturing Wellness: The Path to Breast Cancer Awareness

The breast has always been the symbol of womanhood and ultimate fertility. As a result, both disease and surgery of the breast evoke a fear of mutilation and loss of femininity.

Breast cancer remains a major health concern due to its high incidence worldwide and the significant impact it has on women's health.

This book contains vital information about the prevalence, prevention and tips for early detection of breast cancer for better survival rates.

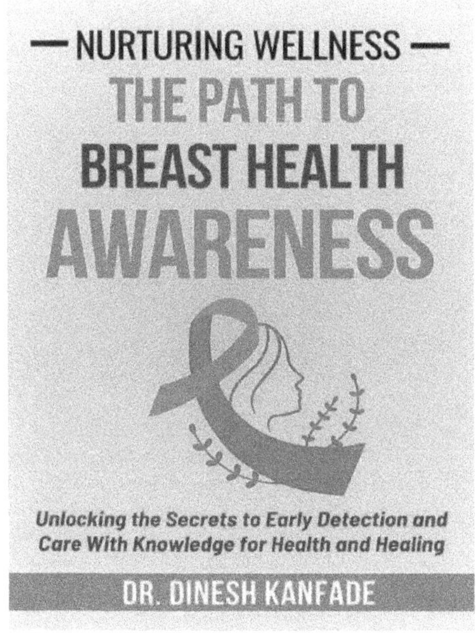

8. Nurturing Wellness: The Path to Postmenopausal Heart Disease Awareness

The biggest achievement of the last century is greater longevity that has resulted in increasing aged population worldwide. It is obvious that women have to live significant part of their lives after menopause. Menopause transition brings profound hormonal changes that can affect multiple aspects of health, including an often-overlooked issue: cardiovascular disease (CVD). Heart disease is the leading cause of death among women in postmenopausal age group, cancer being second. Yet many women are unaware of the heightened risk of CVD they face after menopause. The benefit of increased lifespan is only when it is translated into healthy aging.

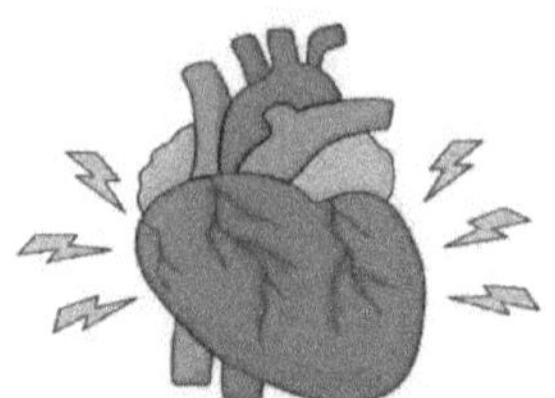

9. Nurturing Wellness: The Path to Postmenopausal Osteoporosis Awareness

Osteoporosis is frequently called the "Silent Killer" because it itself has no symptoms. The patients are unaware of their bone loss until they experience a fracture.

With aging, bone density naturally decreases in both genders, but for many women, this process accelerates after menopause due to estrogen deficiency, leading to brittle bones, subsequent fractures, and a significant impact on quality of life. Despite its widespread prevalence, osteoporosis remains an often-overlooked health issue, overshadowed by other conditions.

The rapid bone loss typically starts within the first 5 - 7 years after menopause, with women losing up to 20% of their bone mass during this period.

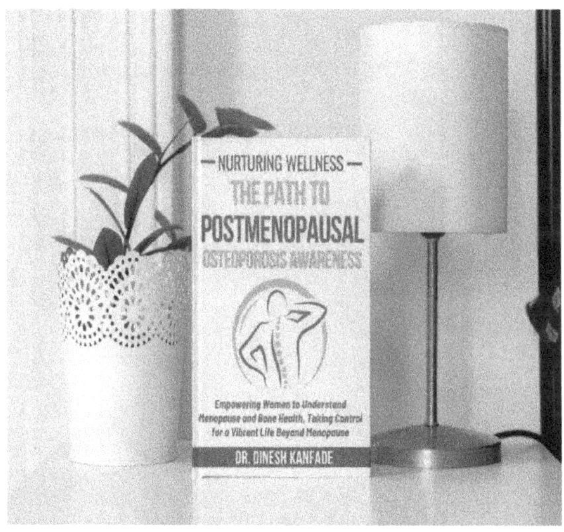

10. Demystifying Menopausal Hormone Therapy

Menopause is a natural phase in every woman's life, yet it often comes with confusion, fear, and unanswered questions—especially regarding hormone therapy. **"Demystified Menopause Hormone Therapy"** is a transformative guide that breaks down the myths and misconceptions surrounding Menopause Hormone Therapy (MHT), offering clear, evidence-based insights for women and medical practitioners alike.

Authored by a seasoned gynecologist, this book delves into the latest research on MHT, addressing its safety, benefits, and practical application. It provides tailored guidance for women with diabetes, hypertension, and other conditions, empowering them to make informed decisions.

Whether you're navigating menopause, supporting a loved one, or offering professional care, this book is your trusted companion in understanding and embracing the journey of menopause with confidence and clarity.

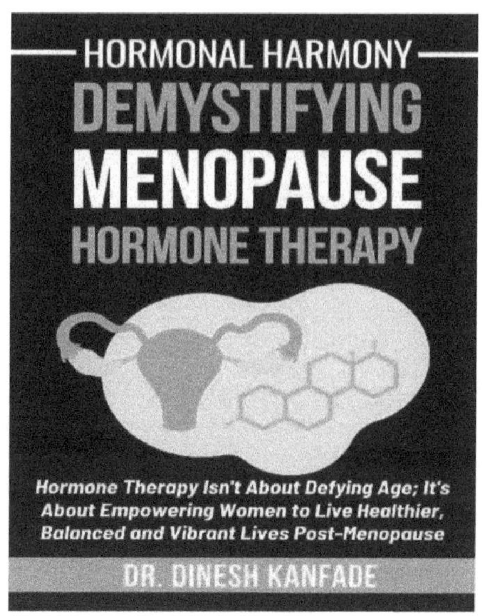

www.ingramcontent.com/pod-product-compliance
Lightning Source LLC
Chambersburg PA
CBHW040800120726
48005CB00012B/1251